Technologies of Life and Death

Technologies of Life and Death

From Cloning to Capital Punishment

Kelly Oliver

FORDHAM UNIVERSITY PRESS

NEW YORK 2013

Library of Congress Cataloging-in-Publication Data

Oliver, Kelly, 1958–
Technologies of life and death : from cloning to capital punishment /
Kelly Oliver. — First edition.
    pages cm
Includes bibliographical references and index.
ISBN 978-0-8232-5108-7 (cloth : alk. paper) —
ISBN 978-0-8232-5109-4 (pbk. : alk. paper)
    1. Bioethics. 2. Biotechnology—Moral and ethical aspects. I. Title.
QH332.O45 2013
174.2—dc23

                                        2012049120

Printed in the United States of America

15 14 13   5 4 3 2 1

First edition

For my dad, who stands by us through thick and thin

CONTENTS

ACKNOWLEDGMENTS

I would like to thank my research assistants over the last several years, Melinda Hall, Juliana Lewis, Alison Suen, and Erin Tarver, who went beyond the call of duty in helping me prepare this manuscript. Thanks to Elissa Marder and Steven Miller for helpful comments on an earlier draft; the book is better for their suggestions. Thanks to Kas Saghafi, organizer of the 2011 Spindel Conference on Derrida and the death penalty, for inviting my participation, which inspired the chapter on animals and capital punishment.

As always, thanks to Benigno, Yuki, Hurri, and Mayo for their companionship.

Technologies of Life and Death

Introduction: Moral Machines and Political Animals

> ... life is the ferocious force that keeps propelling us,
> at the same time, you can just pierce it and it dies.
>
> — KIKI SMITH, 1991

With advances in technoscience, it becomes increasingly difficult to distinguish nature from culture, the grown from the made. Geneticists can enhance the DNA of almost any living creature, including human beings. Cloning is a reality, no longer just the stuff of science fiction. New genetic engineering and organ transplantation technologies raise legal questions about the ownership of one's own DNA and one's own body. Who has the right to reproduce certain DNA, particularly if some DNA (disease resistant) is more desirable than other DNA (disease prone)? In laboratories, we can reproduce most things living and dead. Technologies of reproduction of everything from genes and organs to YouTube videos and the complete works of Shakespeare are at the forefront of our contemporary world. Technology is changing what we mean by *reproduction* itself. Virtually every facet of our lives is mediated by technology, from conception and birth—which can involve drug treatments, high-tech fertility treatments, and

1

planned C-sections—to old-age and death—which usually involve medical and pharmaceutical interventions, if not also pacemakers and other artificial body parts. Of course, along with these new technologies come new ethical and political concerns, issues that affect fundamental questions of life and death. In this book, I examine some of the ways that technology, from cloning to capital punishment, raises ethical and political questions at the extremes of life, namely, at birth and death.

Technological advances give the impression that we are finally about to unlock the secrets of life and death. We feel on the verge of decrypting and decoding the "program" that is life itself. The seeming miracles of modern science give us the sense that eventually we will know with certainty the answers to all of our questions about our own bodies, our place in evolution, and our genetic futures. Some scientists and bioethicists believe that in the very near future we will be able to master our own destinies, perhaps even double, or more than double, our lifespans. Here, I analyze and challenge this *will to mastery* as it appears in discourses of birth and death. In some sense, birth and death are the most certain parts of our lives: we are all born and we all die. But, given advances in assisted reproductive technologies and cloning, can we be certain that we know what it is to be born? And even technological advances have not assured us that we know what it is to die. Birth and death are two experiences—if they *are* experiences—we never witness for ourselves. In a significant sense, we are not present at our own births. And we have yet to hear the testimony of anyone who has reported back from death—near-death perhaps, but not death as such. These are two inevitabilities for every human being, and yet we are still far from unlocking their secrets, from decoding their codes, deciphering their ciphers, or decrypting their crypts. There is always something that escapes us, something in excess of our theories or religions, something that remains inaccessible. And new developments in technology that purport to shed light on reproduction or birth and promise a pain-free death at the same time make all the more vivid how little we know about the beginnings or ends of life. It is as if we are in the dark, trying to invent scopic technologies that enhance our vision so that we can subject birth and death to scientific examination; but, inevitably, regardless of advances in technology, what we see is that there is always more that we cannot see, more to be seen, another dimension, a smaller particle, another galaxy, a new element heretofore unknown. From a philosophical perspective, even as we "find" new particles, galaxies, and elements, these "facts" tell us very little about the *meaning* of life or of death. Furthermore, we might ask, how does technology change what we *mean* by birth or by death?

In philosophy, debates over genetic engineering, cloning, and assisted reproduction, along with discussions of technologies that promise to provide painless humane death, particularly in the context of capital punishment, are dominated by analytic philosophy. Most are framed by the assumption that we can distinguish nature from culture, the grown from the made, the original from the copy. Most such discussions also involve assumptions about liberal autonomous individuals making free and rational choices about their use of these technologies—or in the case of condemned persons, assumptions about their having given up the right to free choice as a result of having broken a contract into which they had implicitly, if not explicitly, entered as citizens of the sovereign state. Issues of sovereignty are central to debates over both cloning and capital punishment. Debates over cloning and genetic engineering often revolve around the question of sovereignty and who has the right to choose. Debates over capital punishment revolve around questions of the sovereignty of the state to decide who lives and who dies.

In this book, I complicate these discussions by introducing Jacques Derrida's challenges to the liberal conception of sovereignty. Developing, extending, and applying his critique, I reframe debates over life and death, from cloning to capital punishment, in the hopes of opening an alternative path through the thickets of these controversies. Throughout his writings, Derrida has insisted on a technological supplement at the heart of everything we have taken to be natural. He has even suggested that technologies of reproduction and the paradoxes they produce may be the fundamental paradoxes of our age (1993). From his earliest work, he has engaged with technologies of reproduction, particularly the reproduction of texts and images. And, from the beginning, machines haunt his texts. The machine appears as a metaphor for technology, certainly; but more than this, it appears as a cipher for the undecidability between original and copy, real and artificial, nature and culture, determinism and freedom, grown and made, chance and choice—the very oppositions that continue to drive debates over reproductive technologies, whether they are genetic or televisual.[1] Derrida spent his career "deconstructing" these oppositions, the very ones that galvanize philosophers, politicians, and religious leaders to "take sides" and declare their opponents irrational, criminal, or worse. One of the ways we can throw a wrench into the binary works is by turning machine against machine, by turning the machine back on itself.

This book uses the deconstructive machine on, and against, the extremes of birth and death insofar as they are mediated by *technologies of life and death*. First, with an eye to reproductive technologies, I consider how the terms of debates over surrogacy, genetic engineering, and cloning change if we use deconstruction machinery to challenge the oppositions that drive them—namely, grown versus made, chance versus choice, and nature versus culture. Next, I consider how art or poetry might provide a counterbalance to political sovereignty, whether state sovereignty or individual sovereignty, when it comes to questions of choosing life or death. Finally, I take up state sovereignty directly with an analysis of the death penalty and capital punishment to show how the scale, scope, and unconscious of sovereignty work to shore up its precarious scaffolding. In conclusion, I consider the tense relationship between the ethical and the political realms as implicated by issues of reproduction of life and of death.

Deconstruction Has Always Been about Cloning

Given that from the beginning Derrida's work has engaged the problematic of reproduction, we could say that deconstruction has always been about cloning. It has always been about the relationship between the so-called original and the copy, whether we are talking about the reproduction of biological material or of a landscape through photography or painting. And, insofar as Derrida identifies an absence at the core of presence, a death at the heart of life, technologies of life are never far from technologies of death.[2]

Although technology and machines are central themes in much of Derrida's corpus, my project here is neither a synthesis nor a catalogue of his machines.[3] This is not a book about Derrida per se; rather it is about how a deconstructive approach can change the very terms of contemporary debates over technologies of life and death, from cloning to capital punishment. Inspired by the deconstruction of sovereignty and of the liberal autonomous sovereign subject in Derrida's last seminars *The Beast and the Sovereign*, volumes 1 and 2 (2009, 2011), I turn to issues raised by our thoroughly technologically mediated contemporary life and death, including concerns surrounding artificial insemination, new reproductive technologies, and technologies of death. Focusing on the extremes of technologically mediated birth and death, I use deconstruction to challenge the liberal individual assumed in most mainstream discussions of these issues to show how tensions in liberal notions of sovereignty not only lead us into theoretical conundrums, but also and moreover may risk leading to war, torture, death chambers, and even genocide.[4]

Here, I analyze technologies of life and death by bringing Derrida into conversation with such thinkers as Jürgen Habermas, John Harris, Julia Kristeva, Immanuel Kant, and Emmanuel Levinas; and I put deconstruction into dialogue with different approaches and methodologies, including liberalism and psychoanalysis, among others. By challenging us to think through the assumptions and fundamental terms of current debates over new reproductive technologies and the beginnings of life, along with those surrounding killing machines that promise clean and painless death, a deconstructive approach combined with psychoanalysis yields a new conceptual field, and thereby reframes the central terms of these discussions and opens up different ways of thinking about them. The central aim of this book is to approach contemporary problems raised by technologies of life and death as ethical issues that call for a more nuanced approach than mainstream philosophy provides. Indeed, as we will see, the ethical stakes in these debates are never far from political concerns such as enfranchisement, citizenship, oppression, racism, sexism, and the public policies that normalize them. In part, then, this book seeks to disarticulate a tension between ethics and politics that runs through these issues, in order to suggest a more ethical politics by turning the force of violence in the name of sovereignty back against itself. In the end, I propose that we bring deconstruction and psychoanalysis together to do so. Deconstructive hyperbolic ethics with a psychoanalytic supplement can provide a corrective for moral codes and political clichés that risk turning us into mere answering machines.

Ethics Machines

Since Nietzsche's proclamation that "God is dead" (and so then are all foundational principles), a central question for philosophy, especially

Continental philosophy, has been how to formulate any sort of normative ethics—that is to say, an ethics that can distinguish right from wrong—after the "deconstruction" of oppositions between good and evil, right and wrong, subject and other, life and death, and so forth (see Nietzsche [1882], section 125). Throughout his writings, Derrida aims his deconstructive strategy—his deconstructive machine—toward these types of oppositions, starting with oppositions between speech and writing, presence and absence, positive and negative, nature and culture, interior and exterior, and ending with oppositions between mind and body, response and reaction, man and animal, and man and God, among many others along the way. Deconstruction is not, however, about collapsing those binaries or demonstrating how good and evil, mind and body, or man and animal are really the same. Rather, it is about showing how these oppositions are too simplistic and cover up complicated and fluid differences within the categories. For example, there is not just one type of man (think of women, the history of humankind, cultural differences, racial differences, etc.), and there is not just one type of animal. This is one of Derrida's most poignant examples; for once we think about it, it is obvious that the category *animal* covers over vast, nearly infinite, differences between species and individuals. Derrida is not trying to abolish the limits between these various oppositions; rather he is attempting to multiply limits, and thereby acknowledge more differences (2008). He describes his approach as a "philosophy of limits."

Throughout his writings, Derrida has invoked various liminal, threshold, and Janus-faced concepts to jam the machinery of binary oppositions so prominent in traditional metaphysics and in philosophy more generally. In *Of Grammatology*, he calls these concepts *nicknames* for the "unnamable movement of difference itself," the operation by which all sameness and "nameness" takes place. Some of his nicknames for this silent operation that he discerns in so many texts of literature, psychoanalysis, and philosophy are *trace, reserve, différance, supplement, dissemination, pharmakon, parergon, hymen, aporia, hospitality, autoimmunity,* and *bêtise,* among many others. Derrida chooses these figures because they have multiple meanings usually at odds with each other. *Animal* and *machine* become such figures.

In *The Animal that Therefore I Am,* Derrida suggests that his concern with animals runs throughout his work; he mentions several texts wherein different animals play central roles, texts he claims he signs in the names of various animals, including hedgehogs and silkworms. But another figure that runs throughout his texts is the machine.[5] There are typewriter ribbons, paper machines, computers, the World Wide Web, word processors, and prosthetic memories and archiving machines of all sorts—indeed prosthesis of all sorts, including wooden legs, marionettes, artificial reproduction technologies, and technologies of reproduction of all sorts, writing machines and writing as a machine, televisions, cameras, printing presses, ink made from the blood of animals, and all varieties of representing machines (e.g., 2009, 2005, 2000b). There are too many machines to list them all here. And then there are the machinations of all of these machines, most especially the machinations of representation, especially of texts (no text without grammar, no grammar without machine, as he says in an essay on Paul de Man's typewriter ribbon), but also the machinations of deconstruction, what he calls "slow and differentiated deconstruction" (2009, 75–76).[6] The *machine*, like the *animal*, can be read as another nickname for the operation of *différance* insofar as it is an undecidable figure or concept that both works for and against the binary oppositions and dichotomies so popular in our culture, most especially nature and culture, body and mind, and animal and man. For, we might ask, which side of the binary is more mechanical?

There are mechanistic operations on both sides of the nature-animal and culture-human divide. It is not just that humans are animals too and our bodies are subject to natural laws; or as scientists may say, that our brains are hard-wired, or that they operate like complicated computer programs. It is not just that there are many ways in which we are like animals or machines in our responses to things, or are even perhaps entirely determined by our DNA or chemical make-up. Rather, culture also operates like a machine that can determine our actions and make what we take to be responses seem more like reactions. For example, everyday greetings— "Hello," "How are you?"—are "programmed" into our behavior. When we think about it, how many of the things that we do are "programmed" by our society and our cultural customs? Even if we believe that at least some of our actions are thoughtful, individual, or unique, how can we be sure where to draw the line between those that are responses and those that are mere reactions? It is not that response and reaction amount to the same thing, or that animals are people too, or that culture operates according to deterministic natural laws. To the contrary, the challenge is to critically reflect on our commonly held beliefs, especially our commonly held assumptions about our own abilities and the lack of those same abilities in others, including animals and machines. In this way, deconstructive ethics multiplies differences and fractures traditional boundaries. Once we wedge the machine in between the binaries animal-human and nature-culture, however, their oppositional stance grinds down, if it does not come to a complete halt.

The invocation of *the machine*, like the invocation of *the animal*, has powerful implications for thinking about ethics and the distinction between morality and ethics (cf. Oliver 2007). When morality becomes a matter of following rules and principles, then it risks becoming mechanical. And, if politics is merely a matter of following laws, then we risk losing sight of justice. So how do we avoid becoming mechanical in our relationship to ethics and to politics? How can we avoid becoming answering machines? I suggest that by acknowledging and examining the mechanisms on both sides of oppositional binaries, even if we cannot stop the machine, or throw a wrench into it, we can turn it back against itself in order to slow it down, even perhaps to open up alternatives. The stakes of doing so are great. The aforementioned conceptual binaries posed as oppositions that beget hierarchies have real-world consequences. For example, the nature-culture divide has played a crucial role in sexism, slavery, genocide, and animal slaughter, among other social concerns that we now consider unjust or wrong.[7] As we know, women, people of color, other religions and cultures, and animals have been relegated to the *nature* side of this divide and variously described as subhuman or barbaric and therefore in need of elimination, discipline, or at least civilizing. The binary logic often brings with it a hierarchy that privileges one side while denigrating the other. This has real-world ethical and political consequences.

By engaging contemporary issues raised by technological advances in administering both life and death, I hope to show not only the applicability of the deconstructive strategy to contemporary debates, but also the necessity of employing it to avoid reducing issues to simple oppositions that elide crucial facets of them. Only by trying to deal with these messy real-life issues in all of their complexities can we hope to think through some of the most pressing ethical and political concerns raised by technologies of life and death. In this book, commonly accepted binaries and concepts important to debates over reproducing both life and death are subjected to the machinations of deconstruction in the hopes of moving beyond the impasses caused by assumptions about nature and freedom, and in order to more realistically access the complexities of these issues as they play out in our lives. While the deconstructive approach does not and cannot provide clear-cut moral guidelines for adjudicating these debates, it does open up new ways of conceiving of the stakes in them; and this opening is necessary for ethics—ethics against moralism—and a more ethical politics.

Answering Machines

In *The Beast and the Sovereign*, Derrida sets out only one rule: "The only rule for the moment I believe we should give ourselves in this seminar is no more to rely on commonly accredited oppositional limits between what is called nature and culture, nature/law, physis/nomos, God, man, and animal or concerning what is 'proper to man' [no more to rely on commonly accredited oppositional limits] than to muddle everything and rush, by analogism, toward resemblances and identities. Every time one puts an oppositional limit in question, far from concluding that there is identity, we must on the contrary multiply attention to differences, refine the analysis in a restructured field" (2009, 15–16). This rule is a rule against rules. It is a rule to question all rules; and furthermore, not to rely on commonly accepted rules, truths, or facts, especially about others that we consider outsiders, enemies rather than friends, or even food rather than intelligent beings. This doesn't mean, however, that we assimilate them and rush to embrace them as really like us after all. Deconstructive ethics, then, is not an ethics of empathy (contrast this to Husserl's analysis of analogical transfer to the place of others through which we know they exist and through which we can empathize with them). Nor is it a moral code or set of moral rules, unless you count the countercommand to question all rules. Deconstruction is not moralism, and if it becomes moralism then it risks re-enacting the very dangers it tries to avoid by vigilantly questioning everything, even its own most cherished principles and ideals.

A deconstructive approach to ethics does not provide a moral code or blueprint that we simply follow to *get it right*. This is not to say that deconstructive ethics does not allow us to take a position on an issue, for example on cloning or the death penalty. Still, we must always be willing to interrogate our own concepts and motives; and in the case of the death penalty, the ways in which we may self-righteously protest against capital punishment while continuing to disavow the ways in which we benefit from other forms of death penalties. Certainly, learning and following rules is easier than having to decide each and every time about what is right and what is wrong. And while we need rules (like the rules of the road and civil laws), following them easily becomes a matter of training or even habit. It is not usually a difficult ethical decision whether or not to stop at a red light, whether or not to say "hello" to an acquaintance on the street, or whether or not to steal, accost, or kill other people. Usually, we merely react to laws and customs without thinking about them, without really responding; we are like machines or trained animals. But unlike moral codes, rules, or civil laws, the difficult ethical choices of our lives are not, and cannot be, so straightforward. They require time, slow and differentiated deliberations, quandaries, even paradoxes, that force us to take our chances, to risk everything we commonly believe or what is commonly accredited.

The hyperbolic command of deconstructive ethics is to hold open the questions of right and good, even if to do so is to risk living on unstable ground when it comes to answering any of the perennial questions of philosophy—questions that Kant formulated as, What can I know? What should I do? What can I hope for? (see Kant 1999, A805/B833). These questions revolve around concerns for ethical life and perhaps an implicit acknowledgment that we cannot separate epistemology (what we know) and metaphysics (what is real) from ethics (what we ought to do), as philosophers are so fond of doing. But, we might ask, without a solid metaphysical ground, how can we begin to answer Kant's questions? Indeed, if the oppositional logics that produce hierarchical thinking, and more to the point, discriminatory or oppressive political regimes, are part and parcel of the history of metaphysics, how can we move beyond it? Can we use the logic of metaphysics against itself in an attempt to designate within the language of philosophy—or we might as well just say within language, period—the impossibility of its own operations, which always escape it? In *Of Grammatology* Derrida says: "Of course the designation of that impossibility escapes the language of metaphysics only by a hairsbreadth. For the rest, it must borrow its resources from the logic it deconstructs. And by doing so, find its very foothold there" (1976, 314). In his later work, however, even that foothold becomes unstable, such that the ground is constantly shifting beneath our feet. In *The Beast and the Sovereign,*

Derrida echoes Gilles Deleuze's formulation that the ground is no more than the dirt stuck to our soles/souls (2009, 151–52).

If we cannot be sure that we know right from wrong, if we cannot be sure that the conventions of our society are just, then we have a radical responsibility to always be on the lookout for injustice, most particularly in those moments or places where we feel most sure of ourselves. Derrida goes so far as asking whether we have an ethical obligation to welcome even those who threaten us (2009, 240). And his analysis suggests that perhaps ethics begins only when we welcome even the most dangerous other. Only when we are willing to risk everything, only then justice may be possible. We have to take our chances, which is not to say we can simply throw the dice or flip a coin in order to decide how to act. Far from it. The chance and risk that Derrida insists are integral to ethics involve the slow and differentiated movements of painstaking critical thinking, of facing the abyss, and only then taking the leap, never once and for all, but over and over again, and never on level ground or with sure footing. Rather than a quick fix, hyperbolic ethics may be a counterbalance to our cultural craving for instant gratification and a quick solution to every problem; we seem to want rules and regimens for everything from losing weight to finding a soul mate, and of course for making money. Deconstructive thinking forces us to slow down and think about the customs and rules that we commonly accept.

Again, we might suppose that challenging our customary ways of thinking about binary oppositions means throwing everything to the wind, including ethics and ethical responsibility for others. But, to the contrary, Derrida insists that deconstructive ethics calls for "a great vigilance as to our irrepressible desire for the threshold, a threshold that is a threshold, a single and solid threshold. Perhaps there never is a threshold, any such threshold. Which is perhaps why we remain on it and risk staying on the threshold for ever" (2009, 333–34). In other words, first we must be attentive to our desire for limits, categories, and fixed boundaries between nature and culture, man and animal, good and evil. And, I would add, we need to be vigilant about when this shows up as a defensive or offensive strategy; and this is where psychoanalysis is useful. Second, we must risk staying on the threshold of undecidability, which is to say, never deciding *once and for all* what/who something is and how we should respond to it/her. Rather, we need to decide each time with slow and differentiated deliberations; and then we need to continue to interrogate our own motives, even unconscious fears and desires, in relation to our answers to all of Kant's questions: what we think we can know, what we think we should do, and what we hope for.

This is why Derrida relentlessly aims his deconstructive approach at some of our most cherished concepts and beliefs—not in order to destroy them, but rather, in a sense, to protect them. He applies his deconstructive machinery against the machinations of oppositional and categorical thinking that lead to violence, war, and genocide in the hopes of preventing the worst of it. Yet the movements of this machine are always precarious and risky because even as the deconstructive machinery is aimed at concepts such as justice, liberty, and democracy, it is also aimed at itself. Derrida articulates this risk as a double bind, the twisting, raveling, and unraveling machinery of deconstruction: "Liberty and sovereignty are, in many respects, indissociable concepts. And we can't take on the concept of sovereignty without also threatening the value of liberty. . . . The double bind is that we should deconstruct, both theoretically and practically, a *certain* political ontotheology of sovereignty without calling into question a certain thinking of liberty in the name of which we put this deconstruction to work" (2009, 301; note that Derrida says a "a *certain* political ontotheology" to indicate that there are various forms). In other words, the goal is not to do away with liberty, freedom, or the nation-state. It is not to do away with sovereignty, or nature—but, rather, to rethink sovereignty outside of a discourse of mastery or even autonomy and towards a more fluid concept that opens up rather than closes off ethical and political questions. The problem is to be vigilant in discerning the ways in which these concepts become the justifications for limiting the freedoms of others, occupying other nations, or generally the rationale for violence, war, and killing.

To make it more concrete, Derrida gives the example of mental asylums and zoos. We want to challenge those institutions in the name of liberty for all and yet not to the point that we have no limits, no walls, no fences, an absolute freedom of movement for everyone; in other words, a world without laws. We want to argue for liberty, but always within limits. No one wants to give up the safe haven of his or her own home, if one is fortunate enough to have one. Deconstruction is not a call for more lock-ups or no lock-ups, more fences or no fences, more laws or no laws, but rather a hyperbolic vigilance in analyzing how these lock-ups, fences, and laws do violence that we disavow, or that we don't want to see, or that we don't see, or perhaps can't even see. The answer, then, is not kinder, gentler lock-ups. Deconstruction is not liberalism. On the contrary, deconstruction challenges liberal discourses of justice, liberty, and democracy to vigilantly attempt to see their own blind spots. This hyperbolic ethics subjects liberal values to the deconstructive machine, not in order to produce alternative moral codes or values, but rather in order to continually feed codes and values into it in the hopes "that the event might challenge or surprise the other machination," the machinations of exclusionary logics that always include some as us or friend and exclude others as them or enemy. It sets us the urgent, impossible, but necessary task of inventing limits that are not lock-ups.

One Nail Takes Out Another

At this point, we might ask, what distinguishes the hyperbolic move of sovereignty from the hyperbolic move of deconstructive ethics? The answer may be that the former leaves no remainder, no excess, while the later insists on exposing it. Hyperbolic sovereignty claims to be the best, the most, indivisible, self-sustaining, and self-sufficient. Hyperbolic ethics, on the other hand, maintains that there is always a remainder, always excess, always another response to give, always another obligation to consider, always an other and otherness upon whom we prop ourselves up. The role of hyperbole in deconstructive ethics is to continually subject the ideal to the double movement. The ideal itself must come under scrutiny for the ways in which it works against itself to create the very thing it claims to prevent. The ideal is a moving target precisely because there is no ideal in itself, but rather concepts that have histories and contexts. *Justice*, *liberty*, and *democracy* are such concepts, concepts in whose name we perpetrate the greatest violence, torture, and war. So too, the concepts of freedom, choice, chance, and nature can be put in the service of justifying violence.

   In *The Beast and the Sovereign*, Derrida is deconstructing the concept—or a *certain* concept—of sovereignty, and more generally the opposition between human (sovereign) and animal (beast). There, Derrida acknowledges that there is no escaping the logic of sovereignty (just as he acknowledges that there is no escaping the metaphysics of presence—the assertion that something *is* such and such). Every time one asserts oneself as a self, as an agent, as someone who can do something, or anything, one is asserting one's sovereignty. The *certain* sovereignty that Derrida has in his sights is one of hyperbole (2009, 257). Toward the end of the seminar, Derrida takes aim at this certain kind of sovereignty that claims to be the *more than*, *the most*: "What is essential and proper to sovereignty is thus not grandeur or height as geometrically measurable, sensible, or intelligible, but excess, hyperbole, an excess insatiable for the passing of every determinable limit: higher than height, grander than grandeur, etc." (257). At first blush, this sounds a lot like the hyperbolic ethics of deconstruction: it is excessive, hyperbolic, insatiable, passing every limit. So, what is the difference between the hyperbolic move of sovereignty and the hyperbolic move of deconstructive ethics? The passage continues: "It [sovereignty] is the *more*, the *more than* that counts, the absolutely more, the absolute supplement that exceeds any comparative toward an absolute superlative" (257).

In this book, combining deconstruction with psychoanalysis, I attempt to disarticulate the concepts of sovereignty, freedom, choice, nature, and culture as they come to play in debates over reproducing life and death, from cloning to capital punishment. Here, I focus on the ways in which deconstruction with a psychoanalytic supplement can assist us in moving through the dense thicket of ethical problems and political dilemmas surrounding technologies of life and death. Along the way, each chapter provides interpretations, perhaps not always orthodox, of some of the most intractable paradoxes of deconstructive ethics, including concepts of purity, hyperbole, generation, witnessing, and mourning, among others. Each chapter shows how one nail takes out another in the history of the philosophy of sovereignty, particularly as that concept plays itself out in contemporary debates over the reproduction of life and of death.

Part I: Sex Machines

In the first chapter, "Genetic Engineering: Deconstructing *Grown* versus *Made*," I use the deconstruction of the nature-culture dichotomy, with its attendant opposition between grown and made, to challenge debates in bioethics over cloning. Indeed, deconstructing the central terms assumed in these debates can change the very framework of them. These debates are currently dominated by the liberal notion of an autonomous individual with free choice, precisely the notion of the sovereign subject that comes under scrutiny in Derrida's later work. Taking John Harris and Jürgen Habermas as representatives of two sides in debates over genetic engineering and cloning, I show how deconstruction unsettles both. In addition, I consider Derrida's own views on cloning and how they might help us navigate complex ethical issues raised by new technologies of reproduction.

In the second chapter, "Artificial Insemination: Deconstructing *Choice* versus *Chance*," I take up Derrida's metaphorical question, "Does one invent the child?" (from the mid-1980s). Given recent advancements in genetic engineering and cloning, this question takes on a more literal hue. So-called designer babies threaten to turn parents into patents in ways that assume we can control reproduction. Derrida's "deconstructive genealogy" presents a challenge to the notion of parent as patent and suggests that even in the face of changing technologies, we cannot control the chance elements of reproduction, even within the most reliable machines. Here, I turn the notions of *parent* and *patent* against themselves, which opens up alternative meanings of both, and again enables one nail to take out another. Furthermore, technologies that raise anew the question of maternity merely highlight the ways in which both maternity and paternity are always uncertain, matters of chance, and assume a problematic notion of testimony. In the end, I argue that current debates in bioethics over genetic engineering assume that we can master reproduction through technologies (whether we approve of that or not) and disavow chance, which is always operative in the machinery of life, particularly in the reproduction of life.

Part II: Medusa Machines

The third chapter, "Girl Powered: Poetic Majesty against Sovereign Majesty," revolves around the role played by the virgin girl in Derrida's *The Beast and the Sovereign*, vol. 1. Derrida suggests that the figure of the girl is between two marionettes, which I interpret as the machine of culture and the machine of nature. Extending Derrida's suggestion, I argue that the virgin girl both erects and undermines sovereign phallic power, which makes her appearance both necessary and threatening to it. Here I begin to discuss a theme that becomes important in my last chapter, namely, the way in which poetic majesty works against sovereign majesty. One *nail* of majesty takes out the other. In the end, I analyze the rhythms of Derrida's style in terms of the temporality of erection and dissemination.

Continuing the discussion of poetic majesty against sovereign majesty, in chapter 4, "Rearview Mirror: Art, Violence, and Sublimation," I turn to Julia Kristeva, particularly the catalogue *Visions capitale* (published in English as *The Severed Heads: Capital Visions*) that accompanied the Louvre exhibit of the same title that she curated, in order to further explore connections between art, violence, and mothers and girls. Taking up questions of the role of art in counterbalancing our violent urges by giving form to fantasies rather than acting on them, I explore Kristeva's account of the transformative power of art. To this end, I engage Kristeva on the relationship between sadomasochistic subjectivity and art to attempt to begin to distinguish between art that enables us to sublimate violence and art that actually incites violence. Can we tell the difference? And if so, how? In this chapter I ask: What distinguishes art as spectacle from art as transformation? As in Derrida's *The Beast*, Medusa makes a central appearance in Kristeva's *The Severed Heads*. In the end, I bring together Kristeva's, Derrida's, and Louis Marin's analyses of the figure of Medusa to complicate connections between art, girls, and sovereignty.

Part III: Death Machines

In the fifth chapter, "Elephant Autopsy: Optic Machinery and the Scale of Sovereignty," I focus on the scene of elephant autopsy in *The Beast and the Sovereign* in order to analyze what Derrida calls "the globalization of the autopsic model" of sovereignty and power. While in the earlier chapters I consider technologies of life, here I consider technologies of death, which are always intimately connected with those of life. Indeed, from his earliest work, Derrida has argued that life is haunted by technologies of death, particularly insofar as technologies of reproduction are also always technologies of death. In other words, the very technologies of life are also technologies of death. This is the fundamental paradox of witnessing and testimony as the reproduction of the irreplaceable, the unique position of the eyewitness. The sovereignty effect and sovereign power require a unique witness, and witnesses to that witness, in a circulation of the gaze that ends in autopsy. Yet, as we will see, there is a blind spot in this sovereign gaze that again is both necessary and unsettling to it, namely the dead eyes of the elephant. Like an elephant who never forgets, Derrida does not let us forget that sovereign power is erected on death, particularly the death of animals, whether the animals with which we share the planet or the animals within ourselves. In conclusion, I try to imagine a witnessing beyond autopsy, a witnessing to and from the other and otherness, a witnessing beyond recognition, witnessing as joy and mourning that might be the nail we need to take out an even more dangerous and painful one, deadly sovereign power.

In chapter 6, "Deadly Devices: Animals, Capital Punishment, and the Scope of Sovereignty," turning to capital punishment exercised on animals, along with Thomas Edison's experimentation on animals that led to the invention of the electric chair, I develop an alternative genealogy of man's moral and legal sovereignty through animal experiments within the penal code. Exploring associations between speculation, spectacle, and the death penalty, I analyze how the animal is central to the history of capital punishment and the sovereignty it secures. If, within the history of philosophy, death and the death penalty have been considered the property of man alone, we will see that the death penalty becomes man's sole property through its exercise on animals. Crucial to the codification of law in modern Europe, the capital punishment of animals proved the scope of Roman law. Thomas Edison's use of animals in the invention of both the electric chair and the first moving images draws an uncanny relationship between spectacle, animals, and the death penalty.

In the last chapter, "Death Penalties: Ethics, Politics, and the Unconscious of Sovereignty," I address the tense relationship between ethics and politics by looking at the case of Troy Davis, an allegedly innocent black man executed in Georgia in September 2011. I begin by analyzing the ways in which two very different thinkers, Kant and Levinas, articulate the tensions between ethics and politics. Moving through Derrida's notion of hyperbolic ethics as a justice to come, I suggest that deconstructive ethics requires that we take responsibility for finding ourselves caught between ethics and politics in the impossible place of respecting the singularity of each life while generalizing principles such that we can live together on the same planet, even if we occupy different worlds. In conclusion, I argue that in order to acknowledge and avow our own investments in violence and death penalties of all sorts, we need a psychoanalytic supplement to deconstructive ethics such that we become responsible not only for what we do or don't do, but also for our unconscious desires and fears that operate as the hidden reasons for those actions.

PART ONE

Sex Machines

Genetic Engineering: Deconstructing *Grown* versus *Made*

The young runner Caster Semenya was propelled into the international media spotlight when she won the women's world championship 800-meter race in Berlin in 2009. Her instant stardom was not the result of her being the fastest runner in the world, but rather because her competitors "accused" her of being a man and not a woman. The eighteen-year-old reportedly asked the president of Athletics South Africa, "Why did you bring me here? . . . No one ever said I was not a girl, but here [in Berlin] I am not" (quoted in Slot 2009). While so-called gender tests were being conducted by an assortment of "experts" to determine whether or not Caster Semenya was female, there was an outcry in the media over a black African girl being subjected to such humiliation. Some called it racist, others called it sexist, and many called it unfair. Evoking the specter of an exotic other, the *New York Times* cited Dr. Maria New, an endocrinologist at Mount Sinai School of Medicine, who compared Semenya to the Bantu, "a group of indigenous South African people, often hermaphrodites, but they do not always have male genitalia" (quoted in Clarey 2009).

In this chapter, I consider what happens to debates over genetic enhancement and cloning when we "deconstruct" the opposition between *grown* and *made* and the notion of freedom of choice that comes with it. Along with the binary *grown* and *made* come other such oppositions at the center of these debates: *chance* and *choice, accident* and *deliberation, nature* and *culture.* To set the stage, I will survey two positions that can act as guideposts in mapping debates over genetic enhancement: John Harris's liberal theory for enhancement, and Jürgen Habermas's communitarian theory against enhancement. In the last section, I consider Derrida's remarks on cloning and extend his analysis in relation to liberal notions of choice versus chance.[1] By deconstructing the oppositions *grown* versus *made* (or *chance* versus *choice,* or *accidental* versus *deliberate*), and *free* versus *determined,* alternative routes through these bioethical thickets start to emerge. Indeed, Castor Semenya may be a lesson in the glorious ambiguities that keep us alive—and occasionally, even well—when we embrace a notion of freedom and choice that acknowledges rather than disavows the ways in which life always exceeds any simple binary oppositions.

In South Africa, the gender tests provoked strong emotions. The South African sports minister, Reverend Makhenkkesi Stofile, "threatened 'third world war' should the IAAF ban Semenya" (Smith 2009). Maclean Winnie Mandela, ex-wife of former president Nelson Mandela, said that "no one had the right to perform tests on 'our little girl' and warned South Africa's news media to be more patriotic 'without insulting one of our own. Use the freedom of press we gave you properly, because we can take it from you'" (Dixon 2009a, A17). Athletics South Africa president Leonard Chuene reportedly said, "You can't say somebody's child is not a girl. You denounce my child as a boy when she's a girl? If you did that to my child, I'd shoot you" (quoted in Dixon 2009, A1). Chuene maintained that "she has not taken any substance to enhance herself artificially . . . her crime is to be born like that. It is a God-given thing." South Africa's team manager echoed this sentiment, saying, "She believes it is a God-given talent and she will exercise it" (quoted in Casert 2009). And one of Semenya's neighbors told the *Today Show,* "We are quite sure she is a girl. No doubts—she wears panties" (quoted in Porter 2009, A35).

Discussing the gender tests conducted by a gynecologist, an endocrinologist, a psychologist, an internal medicine specialist, and an "expert on gender," bioethicist Alice Dreger said, "[G]enes, hormones and genitals are pretty complicated. . . . There isn't really one simple way to sort out males and females. Sports require that we do, but biology doesn't care. Biology does not fit neatly into simple categories, so they do these tests. And part of the reason I've criticized the tests is that a lot of times, the officials don't say specifically how they're testing and why they're using that test." Dreger claimed that the doctors could examine genes, gonads, genitalia, hormone levels, and medical history, "but at the end of the day, they are going to have to make a social decision on what counts as male and female, and they will wrap it up as if it is simply a scientific decision. . . . And the science actually tells us sex is messy." "Humans like categories neat," said Dreger, "but nature is a slob" (quoted in Clarey 2009, B13).

After the testing board concluded that Semenya could keep her medals but did not publicly comment on whether or not she was female, sports minister Stofile said, "[I]n my view, Caster Semenya's future is in her hands. She can decide to run as a woman, which she is" (quoted in Longman 2009). Commenting on this seemingly paradoxical remark, Judith Butler points out that it suggests both that Semenya can decide on her sex/gender and that she cannot decide because she simply "*is* a woman."[2] Semenya's coach, Michael Seme, also made an ambiguous remark in response to the ruling, saying that Semenya "is going to compete as a woman and will remain a woman until she dies," again suggesting that she has a choice about whether or not to compete or remain a woman (quoted in Longman 2009).

Certainly, the case of Semenya calls into question any fixed notions of natural sex or cultural gender; moreover, it challenges the opposition between them. What is natural? In some sense, it seems that Semenya's gender remains undecidable. If it takes a panel of experts to decide issues of sex or gender, that is because it is far from obvious, as commonly believed. Given that the panel included not only scientists but also sociologists, even the experts seem to agree that sex is not decided by biology or genetics alone. So the question of Semenya's gender includes the issue of who decides and why—becoming as much a political or cultural question as a biological or natural one.

What is cultural? In addition to the already complex relationship between nature and culture or sex and gender, our thoroughly technologically mediated world makes distinctions we once thought obvious more problematic than ever before. It is ironic perhaps that in debates over the most high-tech advances in reproductive technology, the opposition between nature and culture, or grown and made, dominates the landscape. Or perhaps the deep commitments to these fixed categories and the cleft between them is a type of anxious reactionary gesture on the part of philosophers who prefer black and white to shades of gray.

Before the controversy over Castor Semenya, there was the case of Andreas Krieger, a formerly female shot-putter named Heidi, and now a married man. Krieger asks, "Who has the right to be judging someone else's gender?" The *Times* (London) reported that Krieger "was born Heidi, but was fed so many steroids by the coaches of the old East Germany sports regime that his body became so masculine that, eventually, after years of soul-searching depression, he decided to have the transformation completed surgically" (Slot 2009, Sports 58). Krieger said that friends and family asked, "What's happening to you? Are you a man or a woman?" (quoted in Slot 2009, Sports 58). Unlike Semenya, who "is going to compete as a woman and will remain a woman until she dies," Krieger competed as a woman, but became a man.

Perhaps even more than that of Semenya, Krieger's case not only blurs the boundary between male and female, but also between nature and artifice: Was Krieger "naturally masculine," or did drugs make her masculine? Was she naturally inclined to be a transsexual or, as the *Times* suggests, did the little blue pills fed to her by her coaches radically change her? Furthermore, we might ask, was she cheating when she won the European women's shot put championship in 1986? And if so, was it because she was naturally endowed with more masculinity than the other women, or because her coaches gave her performance-enhancing drugs, or both? In other words, was her cheating natural or man-made? And, perhaps more to the point, is her gender—or Castor Semenya's, or anyone's—natural or man-made? This raises more general questions about the relationship between nature and culture, even as they play out in biological sciences that are thought to operate according to set laws. Along with raising strong emotions, the cases of Krieger and Semenya raise philosophical questions over how we draw lines between seeming opposites in order to avoid ambiguities that our culture finds unacceptable, even abject. Here, the categories in question include male and female, nature and artifice, fair and unfair, or cheating. Metaphysical questions of how we separate nature from culture—so-called God-given talent from artificial enhancement—bleed into ethical questions of fair play and cheating. With Semenya, gender—or womanliness—becomes a cipher for both the real and the just.

Grown *versus* Made, *or* Nature *versus* Culture

The distinctions between natural and man-made, God-given and artificial, and fairness and cheating are also at the center of debates over genetic engineering. For example, British philosopher John Harris endorses what he calls *enhancing evolution*, and he talks of "natural selection versus deliberate selection," or "Darwinian evolution versus enhancement evolution" (e.g., Harris 2007, 4). German philosopher Jürgen Habermas insists on the moral relevance of the distinction between "grown versus made," (Habermas 2003, ch. 4). And the American authors of *From Chance to Choice* discuss "normal species functioning" versus enhanced functioning (Buchanan et al. 2000; cf. Harris 2004). Many of these philosophers compare genetic enhancement to artificial enhancements used by athletes. For example, speaking of genetic enhancements, Michael Sandel claims: "The real problem with genetically altered athletes is that they corrupt athletic competition as a human activity that honors the cultivation and display of natural talents" (Sandel 2004). The irony is that in Semenya's case, her "natural talents" have made her competitors and officials suspicious of her "unnatural" natural genetic endowments. These folks feel that the nature of Semenya's "God-given" body threatens to corrupt fair athletic competition.

A further irony is that the libertarian eugenics advocated by philosophers such as Harris could very well lead to a future without a Caster Semenya or a Heidi Kreiger. If their talent is the result of so-called abnormal or defective genes, then gene therapy could "correct" them before birth, while embryo selection could insure that people with their so-called defects are never born. Much of the debate over enhancing evolution revolves around giving some people an unfair advantage over others by enhancing nature. In the cases of Semenya and Kreiger, nature or natural selection gave them what some consider an unfair advantage that deliberate selection could prevent. Alternatively, and equally ironically, given our cultural obsession with sports and celebrity, we might imagine that genetic enhancement may allow parents to choose to alter their daughter's genetic code to make her into a gold medal winner. In other words, we could deliberately tinker with genes in order to produce a more muscular, faster woman—perhaps something like a shot-putting Barbie, with all the strength and speed of a man but without the facial hair.

Most philosophers discussing genetic engineering, including cloning, assume the grown-versus-made opposition. Therefore, their stance on the ethics of both revolves around whether they privilege one side of this binary over the other. Part and parcel of the grown-versus-made opposition is the liberal notion of freedom of choice also assumed in these discussions. Most philosophers engaged in debates over genetic engineering and cloning begin with some version of a liberal sovereign individual who has freedom of choice that must be protected, whether we are talking about the parents' freedom (or lack thereof) in considering genetic engineering and embryo selection, or the future person's freedom (or lack thereof) resulting from such a process. The central question in these debates is whose freedom is most important and thus who gets to exercise their free choice, and why. Although philosophers have different answers to this question—Harris opts for protecting parents' rights to choose, Habermas for protecting the rights of future persons, and some feminists (e.g., Mahowald and Purdy) for guaranteeing women's rights to reproductive choice—all of them assume a sovereign individual, operating either within a social situation that makes them also interdependent, or on an abstract level preferred by some philosophers to avoid the mess of the real world in favor of moral purity.[3]

Controlling the Mess of Nature: *John Harris's* Enhancing Evolution

In *Enhancing Evolution: The Ethical Case for Making Better People* (2007), John Harris echoes his earlier claims in *On Cloning* (2004) that there is an ethical case for "interventions in the *natural lottery of life* and in the course of evolution" (2007, 31; my emphasis). Throughout both books, he argues for making what he calls "better people" by using genetic enhancements as a way to "avoid the risk of the *genetic roulette* that is sexual reproduction and opt for a tried and tested genome of proven virtue" (127, my emphasis; cf. 2004, 29–30). Harris prefers neat categories and moral abstractions that avoid the mess of life, particularly its risks. Harris is not a gambler, and hopes that through genetic enhancement we can avoid the lotteries and roulettes of life. For Harris, whereas natural evolution is a game of chance, deliberate evolution is a game of mastery. Moreover, for Harris, mastery is not only better than chance, but is also the basis for responsibility: "I am master of my fate if I *can* choose, not only if I *do* choose. . . . We cannot escape that burden by declining the *recognition* of our mastery of our fate or by choosing not to make decisions rather than making them in a particular way" (2007, 118; emphases in original).

Harris defines *better* as better able to do things (2007, 2); and, although he concludes that we have an ethical obligation to make ourselves better, he never considers whether or not genetic enhancement will or can make ethically or morally better people. Like most liberal theorists, Harris values individual freedom and choice over what we might call ethical concerns about making people better rather than making better people. Indeed, his analysis turns on a slippage between making people better, in the sense of treating diseases and illnesses through genetic "correction"—or what in this debate is called *negative eugenics*—and making better people through enhancements, or *positive eugenics*.[4] Making people better easily slides into making better people; and he defines *better* in terms of greater ability to compete physically and intellectually, which may even be at odds with what we might consider ethical or moral improvement. Against other theorists (such as Michael Sandel, Leon Kass, and Jürgen Habermas), Harris argues that there is no clear delineation between manipulating genes for therapy (negative eugenics) and for enhancement (positive eugenics).

Harris insists that he is considering all and only morally relevant considerations, which in effect means that he excludes and/or discounts historical, social, and political factors as accidental to any discussion of whether or not enhancing evolution is moral, even morally obligatory. Racism, sexism, homophobia, and other forms of discrimination that not only could, but very likely would, affect so-called freedom of choice in genetic enhancement are considered "contingent" harms that have no bearing on the ethics of enhancement itself (cf. Oliver 2010). For example, in his discussion of the moral neutrality of gender, in passing he dismisses the whole history of women's oppression, saying: "Men and women have existed since humans have and although there have been severe power imbalances between two genders for most of human history, the damage that this has caused is contingent, not a necessary part of maleness or femaleness" (157–58). He argues that since it is not morally better to be a male or a female, it is not morally better to create a male or a female; in other words, gender is morally neutral. He insists that if it isn't wrong to wish for a girl child, then it is not wrong to select for a girl child (2007, 145). What are we to make, then, of the parenthetical remark with which he concludes his argument? "The choice of phenotypical traits such as hair, eye and skin color, physique, stature, and gender are examples of what I call morally neutral choices in the sense that it is not in most circumstances better or worse, morally speaking, to be black, white, tall, short, male or female, brown-haired or blond (*despite what gentlemen allegedly prefer*)" (7, my emphasis).[5] The parenthetical remark with which he ends this passage is symptomatic of the blindness of liberal theory to social and political factors that cannot but affect the morals, freedom, and choice that they hold dear. His humor is born out of sexist stereotypes that not only affect our conceptions of gender and sexual difference, but also affect our supposedly free and sovereign choices. All of our choices are made within the realm of contingency that Harris evacuates from morality. The liberal morals that he endorses, then, are empty insofar as they are based on purely abstract notions of freedom.

While the moral neutrality that Harris assumes in terms of gender is out of step with real moral problems in the social and political world in which we actually live, his insistence on the moral neutrality of race is even more jarring, given ongoing and systematic racism in this country. Again, when we look at his metaphors and his examples, Harris's text betrays him. For example, he uses the metaphor "a whiter shade of pale" when talking about the relative merits on one proposal over another, even when those proposals would most likely have racist implication in the actual world, if not in his ideal world (2007, 113). In addition, at one point he gives an example of genetically engineering people with darker skin to protect against the sun's rays, without considering the politics of darkness and lightness that his metaphorics recalls (2007, 92). His claims to moral neutrality become more strikingly problematic when we substitute race for gender or for disability (which is the issue he uses most often). Consider his claim that if it isn't wrong to wish for a girl child, it isn't wrong to select for one. Now, consider the political situation that might lead black women or black couples to wish for a white child. Of course it is not morally wrong to be black or to be white, but within our culture being white is usually a distinct advantage, and giving our children the advantage and the competitive edge is what it is all about for Harris. As Camisha Russell points out, black women do choose whiter babies, and white women sue if they are mistakenly inseminated with black sperm (cf. Oliver 2012). So, even if race and gender are morally neutral, they are not politically neutral. And, until they are, we cannot so easily separate ethics or morals from politics. Moral norms are political, something Harris and other liberal theorists disavow even while their own language betrays them.

Even on his own terms, there is a fundamental inconsistency in Harris's argument. On the one hand, he rejects appeals to some inherent value in humanity or human nature that we have an obligation to preserve (á la the positions of Sandel and Kass); and on the other hand, his case for liberal freedom of choice is based on his endorsement of freedom as an essential part of humanity or human nature and therefore a basic fundamental right (á la Ronald Dworkin). Harris does not effectively get around the fact that this basic fundamental right is *either* groundless or a matter or consensus and is therefore "up for grabs," so to speak, *or* it is grounded in a notion of nature that he otherwise rejects. In other words, he argues for the freedom of choice in reproduction and genetic enhancement using terms that he has already rejected in favor of better people and a new species beyond humanity or human nature. As an analytic philosopher, he cannot have it both ways.

Harris embraces a new species beyond humanity. He says: "This possibility of a new phase of evolution in which Darwinian evolution, by natural selection, will be replaced by a deliberately chosen process of selection, the results of which, instead of having to wait the millions of years over which Darwinian evolutionary change has taken place, *will be seen and felt almost immediately* [my emphasis]. This new process of evolutionary change will replace *natural selection* with *deliberate selection, Darwinian evolution* with *'enhancement evolution'*" (2007, 3–4). But why, then, are we to believe that this new species will cling to old human conceptions of freedom and choice? Won't our very conceptions of ourselves as free, sovereign individuals also evolve? Perhaps this new species of *Übermenchen* will not see life or evolution in terms of chance versus choice.

If Harris is right that deliberate selection could mean that instead of taking millions of years, changes in our species will be almost immediate, then our sense of time, history, and the concept of evolution itself will be radically changed. Our quest for speed and immediacy will affect us on a genetic level and will hasten evolution to the point that perhaps it will no longer be considered evolution. Certainly, if we develop the ability to create human beings in laboratories without women gestating them or giving birth to them, and combine this with new forms of birth control that do away with menstruation altogether, we may also do away with what Julia Kristeva describes as the monumental and cyclical nature of women's experience of time, along with the sensitivity and creativity of mothers, which makes them, as Kristeva suggests, our only safeguard against producing human beings in laboratories (2002, 402); and what Iris Young describes as the "temporality of movement, growth, and change" of pregnancy and the "timelessness" of labor and birth may disappear (Young 1990, 167). Indeed, what Harris imagines in terms of enhancing both evolution and freedom of choice over chance values linear time, with its clear-cut cause and effect, over other experiences of temporality. In addition, Harris buys into the assumption that faster is better, a notion that has been with us since at least the nineteenth century.

Even if, as Harris imagines, genetic engineering can design new human beings (or a new species beyond the human) in the time it takes to surgically alter embryos—mere nanoseconds compared with the time of Darwinian evolution—he does not consider that for the present, at least, women are still required to gestate babies for nine months and give birth to them through labor that can last days in clock time, but that can be experienced as timeless by the women going through it. Harris's movement between the immediacy of evolutionary changes and his fantasy that these changes may lead to immortality, as we design people who can live without disease forever, collapses the time of life or lived time into the timelessness of the nanosecond or instant—the now of the genetic intervention—and the timelessness of eternal life. What disappears from this fantasy is the time of our lives, the time of contingencies that necessarily interrupt any neat linear cause-and-effect sense of time. Harris's dream of instant immortality condenses the time of evolution and the evolution of time into the now of instant gratification demanded by consumers in a digital age in which the global marketplace is open and operating 24/7, and goods and services can be delivered almost instantly. This instantaneous time, this immediacy resists critical thinking by rendering reflection an inefficient waste of time in a culture that prefers to "just do it" rather than to think about it.

Speeding up evolution may give us "better people" in the sense that they will score higher on IQ tests, jump higher, run faster, and conform better to normalized standards of beauty. But as our science fiction fantasies also imagine, smarter, stronger people or beings are not necessarily morally better; they may not be more altruistic, more compassionate people. Indeed, the value that Harris places on speed, efficiency, and control in evolution seems at odds with a notion of ethics defined as the good life, a prerequisite for which is thoughtfulness and taking one's time. We could say that the temporality of ethics is at odds with the instantaneous time of enhanced evolution imagined by Harris. As we will see, what Derrida calls *hyperbolic ethics* can operate as a counterbalance to the tendency of contemporary culture to act without thinking and to turn morality into a set of regulations and rules for the management of life.

Ethics of the Species: Jürgen Habermas's The Future of Human Nature

In his discussion of genetic enhancement, Jürgen Habermas presents a radically altered notion of the sovereign free individual, embraces the contingencies of life, and strongly disagrees with Harris's conclusions, and yet he too ignores feminism and women's experiences of reproductive choice. He does quote Hannah Arendt on her concept of natality, and he systematically, if not consciously, alternates between using masculine and feminine pronouns when discussing human beings in general. In this regard, at least, his style signals a feminist sensibility. Yet this style also yields unsettling moments for a feminist reader, as when his use of the feminine pronoun to represent the abstract human person displays the awkwardness of that move. In other words, there are moments in his text that make us aware of how "she" does *not* occupy the privileged position Habermas so diligently assumes for her. For example, when describing human freedom and agency, he says:

> [I]t is the person *herself* who is behind her intention, initiatives, and
> aspirations. . . . The capacity of being oneself requires that the person be at
> home, so to speak, in her own body. . . . [I]t compels us to differentiate between
> actions we ascribe to ourselves and actions we ascribe to others. But bodily
> existence enables the person to distinguish between these perspectives only on
> the condition that she identifies with her body. And for the person to feel one
> with her body, it seems that this body has to be experienced as something
> natural. . . . The person, irrespective of her finiteness, knows herself to be the
> irreducible origin of her own actions and aspirations. (2003, 57–58)

To be generous, from a feminist perspective Habermas could be describing an ideal situation; but he is certainly not describing the actual situation of many women in relation to their own bodies. If he were, why would eating disorders and cosmetic interventions be more common in women and girls than in men and boys? Think too of the pregnant body, never mentioned, but always lurking behind these abstract discussions of reproductive choice. Can the pregnant woman identify with her body as her own and feel one with it in the way that Habermas describes? Various feminists and women philosophers have said she cannot. For example, Kristeva suggests that the pregnant subject is emblematic of the split or fragmented subjectivity of all speaking beings and signals the life of speaking beings on the threshold of nature and culture: "[A] woman as mother would be, instead, a strange fold that changes culture into nature, speaking into biology. Although it concerns every woman's body, the heterogeneity that cannot be subsumed in the signifier nevertheless explodes violently with pregnancy (the threshold of culture and nature) and the child's arrival" (1976a, 259). And Iris Young has powerfully articulated what she takes to be a phenomenology of the body of the pregnant woman as "doubled" and "split": "She experiences her body as herself and not herself. Its inner movements belong to another being, yet they are not other, because her boundaries shift. . . . [T]he lived pregnant body . . . challenges [the] implicit assumptions of a unified subject" (1990, 160–61). Going beyond Kristeva, Young argues that what she calls the porosity and openness of pregnant embodiment could be an ethical model for all relationships.

Unlike Harris, Habermas is not oblivious to this type of ethical concern, namely the relationality of all human individuals. In fact, he begins *The Future of Human Nature* by warning of the shortcomings of Rawls's political liberalism, founded as it is on an individualism that separates justice from morality, or at least from ethics understood in the classical sense of "the right way to live" (2003, 2–3). Habermas argues that such theories "may be very good at explaining how to ground and apply moral norms; but they still are unable to answer the question of why we should be moral *at all*" (2003, 4). This problem is implicit, if not explicit, in my earlier engagement with Harris, who can give reasons for genetic enhancement based on individual freedom only by excising from his discussion any broader questions about meaning and justice. Harris can defend the morality of his position only by discounting ethical concerns. We might say that his moral reasoning is possible only by forsaking the ethical altogether.

Habermas turns to Kierkegaard for an alternative conception of freedom that entails very different notions of the individual and of ethics from those assumed in traditional liberal discourse. Interpreting Kierkegaard, Habermas says:

> [The ethically resolute life] demands that I gather myself and detach myself from the dependencies of an overwhelming environment, jolting myself to the awareness of my individuality and freedom. Once I am emancipated from a self-induced objectification, I also gain distance from myself as an individual. . . . In the social dimension, such a person can assume responsibility for his or her own actions and can enter into binding commitments with others. In the temporal dimension, concern for oneself makes one conscious of the historicity of an existence that is realized in the simultaneously interpenetrating horizons of future and past. (2003, 6)

Habermas grounds this interpretation of Kierkegaard on a passage from *Either/Or* in which Kierkegaard seemingly deconstructs the distinction between essential and accidental upon which the morality of liberalism, even of the Habermasian variety, is based. Here is the passage he quotes: "Everything that is posited in his freedom belongs to him essentially, however accidental it may seem to be. . . . [T]his distinction is not a product of his arbitrariness so that he might seem to have absolute power to make himself into what it pleased him to be . . . . To be sure, the ethical individual dares to employ the expression that he is his own editor, but he is also fully aware that he is responsible, responsible for himself personally . . . responsible to the order of things in which he lives, responsible to God" (Kierkegaard, quoted in Habermas 2003, 7). Habermas's immediate focus in reading this passage is on God and Kierkegaard's criticisms of the corruption of Christianity that he witnessed in his society. Eventually, however, his discussion leads him to Kierkegaard's rejection of "an ego-centered consciousness" and the power of reason or will to accept responsibility only by avoiding it, that is, by disavowing its dependence upon an Other as the ground of freedom (cf. 2003, 9). I am sympathetic to Habermas's secular interpretation of this Other as language and meaning rather than as a Christian God. I agree with him when he says "the logos of language embodies the power of the intersubjective, which precedes and grounds the subjectivity of speakers. . . . The logos of language escapes our control, and yet we are the ones, the subjects capable of speech and action, who reach an understanding with one another in this medium" (2003, 10–11). What is missing from his account, and ultimately from what he takes away from Kierkegaard, however, is the element of nonmeaning that resists under-standing that is the heart of language and communication. Again, I agree when Habermas says, "No one possesses exclusive rights over the common medium of the communicative practices we must intersubjectively share. . . . How speakers and hearers make use of their communicative freedom to take yes-or-no positions is not a matter of their subjective discretion. For they are free only in virtue of the binding force of the justifiable claims they raise toward one another" (2003, 10). Where I disagree is in the assumption that claims can be justified and adjudicated using reason alone, and/or once and for all.

Habermas argues that Kierkegaardian ethics "runs up against its limits . . . as soon as questions of a 'species ethics' arise. As soon as the ethical self-understanding of language-using agents is at stake *in its entirety*, philosophy can no longer avoid taking a substantive position" (2003, 11). What Habermas is arguing is that in light of advances in biology and biotechno-logies, neither the liberal position nor the existentialist position can maintain its commitment to "pluralism of worldviews" (cf. 11). Later, I will return to the passage from Kierkegaard to explain why I think that the existentialist path, with its difficulties and despair, gives us greater hope for an ethics than either liberal theory or Habermas's "species ethics." For now, let's continue with Habermas's line of thought.

Given that Habermas is walking the line between communitarian ethics and liberalism, perhaps we should not be surprised that the next philoso-pher he quotes at length is Ronald Dworkin. In "Playing God: Genes, Clones, and Luck," Dworkin argues against genetic enhancement, not in terms of specific moral norms or reasons that might be broken, but rather in terms of breaking the very possibility of morality itself (2000, 427–52). Dworkin concludes that the structure of morality "depends, crucially, on a fundamental distinction between what we are responsible for doing or deciding, individually or collectively, and what is given to us, as a back-ground against which we act or decide, but which we are powerless to change. . . . That crucial boundary between chance and choice is the spine of our ethics and our morality. . . . The popularity of the term 'genetic lottery' itself shows the centrality of our conviction that what we most basically *are* is a matter of chance not choice" (2000, 443–45).

Habermas agrees with Dworkin that the possibility of morality is at stake in genetic enhancement. He argues that our self-understanding as moral beings is intimately and inherently linked to what he calls "the anthropological background of an ethics of the species," by which he seems to mean an ethics based on recognizing ourselves and each other as "responsible authors of our own life history" and of equal dignity with others of our species (2003, 29). At this point, we might wonder how he can invoke the anthropology that grounds species ethics in relation to reproduction without considering the work of feminists, particularly Simone de Beauvoir, whose anthropology of reproduction and "the second sex" transformed the way that we conceive of sexual difference. From the perspective of anthropology, human reproduction, as Beauvoir argues, is governed by various cultural taboos placed on women's bodies, particularly pregnant bodies: "[T]he body of woman is one of the essential elements in her situation in the world. But that body is not enough to define her as woman" (1949, 37); and "It is not merely as a body, but rather as *a body subject to taboos*" (36; my emphasis) that a subject is conscious of him- or herself. We cannot ignore that women give birth and men don't and the ways in which this biological fact has been interpreted and interpolated in human practices of reproduction. Moreover, we cannot disavow, as many in these debates do, that with genetic engineering and cloning, women are and will be required still to gestate and give birth to offspring, even those conceived in laboratories. Anne O'Byrne reminds us that clones will be born and therefore "natal" too: "We were all gestated in the body of another, and it will be no different for the clone, who will not be a 'homunculus in a retort' any more than test-tube babies are born out of test tubes" (2010, 162; cf. Oliver 2012).

In addition to the absence of any account of sexual difference as it relates to the reproduction of the human species upon which Habermas grounds his species ethics, there is little in his text to justify what some might consider the speciesism of his approach and his return to an outdated humanism. Habermas and other philosophers (e.g., Kass) contributing to debates over genetic enhancement appeal to the uniqueness of human beings among other species as a reason for preserving them over all others. The argument from uniqueness, however, can be applied to any animal or plant species as a reason to preserve them from extinction. Moreover, while the human species may be uniquely rational and moral (at least from our own perspective), as a species we are also capable of irrationality and immorality that is more deadly and dangerous to ourselves and other species than the "irrationality" and "immorality" of any other species on the planet. Elsewhere, following Derrida's deconstruction of the man-animal opposition and of the claims to human exceptionalism, I have argued that the conceptual distinction between human beings and other beings fundamental to the history of philosophy does not hold up under philosophical scrutiny (Oliver 2010).

For Habermas, the combination of responsibility and dignity definitive of our species is the foundation of the moral community and of the possibility of ethics, without regard for sexual difference or differential relations to procreation and the reproduction of the species. Habermas maintains that questions of genetic enhancement of embryos is not a question of the moral norms of one culture or group versus the moral norms of another; rather, he argues that the questions of identity raised by this technology touch on "those intuitive self-descriptions that guide our own identification *as human beings*—that is, our self-understanding as member of the species" (2003, 39). If, as Harris suggests, enhancing evolution may give rise to another species of beings beyond the human, then it may also give rise to another species of morality or ethics beyond the human, and perhaps beyond good and evil altogether. This is what worries Habermas. The risk of no longer being able to even identify evil, let alone prevent it, is too high.

Habermas suggests that there is a necessary relationship between contingency and ethics that will be lost with genetic enhancements. If we are made and not grown, as he says, we will not be able to claim our freedom in Kierkegaard's sense of making our lot our own, of embracing what Harris calls the lottery of natural selection. Rather, according to Habermas, their parents will have determined the future people created through genetic engineering. He argues that this generational and irrevocable decision making on behalf of future persons limits their freedom. He distinguishes negative eugenics (correcting a defect or preventing a disease) from positive eugenics (enhancing intelligence or athletic abilities) by invoking a notion of *counterfactual consent* that he claims is available in the first and lacking in the second. In other words, presumably future generations would consent to genetic manipulation of themselves as embryos to prevent a disease, but they could not consent to enhancement, particularly enhancement that makes them different persons, such that the absent persons never existed and therefore could neither consent nor refuse. For Habermas, the freedom of choice of future generations is at stake, along with the ethics of the species, which is based on our freedom to make our own ways in a world full of contingencies. The presumption, which is consistent with liberalism, is that if we are not free to make our own choices, then we are not responsible.

But this sentiment seems to miss the point of Kierkegaard's refusal of the distinction between the essential and the accidental in the face of responsibility. Recall the passage from *Either/Or* quoted by Habermas that begins: "Everything that is posited in his freedom belongs to him essentially, however accidental it may seem to be" (2003, 7). Kierkegaard suggests that whether our existence is essential or accidental, determined or arbitrary, we are responsible, not only to ourselves and to future generations, but also to all others and to the environment that sustains us. Kierkegaard's notion of radical responsibility that results from the refusal of the opposition between the necessary and the contingent challenges both Harris's and Habermas's world views. From this Kierkegaardian perspective, we cannot evacuate what Harris chooses to call contingent aspects of our existence and identities, such as race and gender; neither can we claim, á la Habermas (or Dworkin), that ethics and freedom are the result of the contingency and randomness of our birth. For we are always both grown and made, and we must take responsibility nonetheless. Still, I appreciate the paradoxical element of the Habermasian-Dworkinian position that the ability to decide and choose our own genetics reduces rather than enhances freedom of choice, while our powerlessness in the face of the contingency of a life out of our control increases it.

In sum, on both sides of debates over genetic engineering and cloning, we see that philosophers assume a liberal notion of the sovereign individual who is free to choose, who can make decisions and control the future. For Harris this is a good thing, while for Habermas it is not. Habermas imagines that genetic enhancement would make us masters of our destiny in such a way as to undermine the contingencies that make us free. Yet, for Habermas, it is the authorship of one's own life and the ownership of one's own body that results in human agency, an authorship and ownership already at odds with the contingency he privileges. If we refuse the sovereign author/owner as our starting point, then the contingency of life (and of morality) is not merely the result of an autonomous agent stuck in a contingent world. Rather, the subject itself cannot, contra Habermas, escape the Other and others to which and to whom it is beholden; its existence is a contingency all the way down to the kernel of its subjectivity and agency. It is not that the subject (perhaps á la Sartre) is battling against a hostile or contingent world that threatens its essential and authentic individuality at every turn. Rather, the battle takes place within the subject—or better yet, constitutes the subject—who cannot be unified or reintegrated because its experience is fundamentally fragmented. Ethical responsibility, then, is neither the result of mastery nor of authorship, but is rather the result of a response to the call from the other/Other.

As we have seen, Harris argues for mastery over the future as an ethical imperative; that is to say, in his view we have an ethical responsibility to make better people through genetic technologies, including cloning. He assumes that we can use our scientific knowledge to control the future of the human species, which is precisely what Habermas finds abhorrent. But only by starting with a notion of human agency as sovereign, as lording over nature, can we come to either of these conclusions. In other words, most of the players in these debates assume that human agency is sovereign and that through scientific knowledge and technology we can control if not completely master our destiny. Derrida's challenge to this notion of human agency as sovereign freedom to decide and master not only undermines the conclusions on both sides of the debate, but also and moreover changes the very terms of the debate.

Deconstruction Was Always about Cloning: Jacques Derrida on Reproduction Machines

Derrida's deconstruction of a "certain sovereignty" (which I discuss in chapter 7) presents a challenge to both Harris's and Habermas's assumptions about human sovereignty as it relates to debates over genetic engineering and cloning.[6] As we have seen, both Harris and Habermas think that genetic engineering technologies will allow doctors or parents to decide who or what future children will be and that these technologies will allow human beings to control their own reproduction. This assumes that we are sovereign agents with some knowledge that enables us to decide and predict the future, in this case the future existence or qualities of human beings. This is a grand idea of sovereignty, what Harris embraces as mastering evolution and Habermas reviles as taking away the freedom of future generations. But would even the most advanced genetic engineers or scientists have the kind of sovereignty imagined in these debates? This is not a question of whether the state of current science gives us the knowledge necessary for such mastery and control, but rather the question of whether or not it is possible to possess it at all, ever.

In light of Derrida's analysis of sovereignty, we must ask what it means to decide on one's future children. We must ask, what is freedom in this context? The question is not the one asked by so many bioethicists, namely, whose freedom is most important? The question is, rather, whether this kind of freedom (a certain grand notion of freedom) is ever or could ever be possible. The question is not whether parents or doctors or children should decide, but rather whether such a decision or such deciding is possible. Derrida addresses this question in various contexts when he challenges the history of philosophy's postulation of a subject or agent who "can," who has certain abilities about which we can be certain. In other words, can we be so sure that genetic engineers possess the kind of mastery over future generations that either Harris or Habermas imagines? Won't the children who result from technological interventions still be plagued with suffering and death like their nontechnological predecessors? And won't parents and children still have to figure out how to negotiate their relationships with one another, no matter what technologies are used?

To imagine the kind of mastery and control assumed by Harris and Habermas (for better or worse), one assumes an illusory kind of sovereignty, evidenced by the fact that many of these debates turn around whether or not human beings should "play God."[7] The idea that human beings are capable of "playing God" suggests an absolute and all-powerful sovereignty of the very sort Derrida deconstructs, most explicitly in *The Beast and the Sovereign*. This is not just any sovereignty, or any liberty or freedom, but rather it is sovereignty imagined as absolute mastery that either enhances our freedom, á la Harris, or curtails it, á la Habermas. Moreover, this notion of sovereignty as mastery assumes that the others who come, the children born of these technologies, are not radically other, but always only products designed by their engineers (this is the premise of several dystopian films about cloning, such as *Moon* and *The Island*). Some arguments against genetic engineering and cloning maintain that like products, human beings will be manufactured according to industry standards that will ensure quality control. It is assumed that this control will make human offspring and human life predictable and accident-free. Again, presumptions about oppositions between free and determined and between chosen and accidental are at the crux of the debates over genetic engineering and cloning. Some philosophers ignore the fact that each child is unique, regardless of how closely his or her DNA resembles that of another human being; even "identical" twins are not identical. And to think that clones will be identical in every way is to underestimate the power of nurture over nature. As we have seen, this is another sticking point in the debates—nature versus nurture, or grown versus made. And it is here that Derrida's deconstruction of those very binary oppositions exerts the most pressure.

Discussing cloning in an interview with Elisabeth Roudinesco, Derrida refuses the opposition between naturalism and constructivism, or what others call the opposition between grown and made: "I would prefer not to let myself get trapped in an alternative between naturalism and constructivism. And I do not consider legitimate any of the numerous conceptual oppositions evoked, presupposed, or taken as firmly established in such an alternative" (2004, 39).[8] Of course, this has been one of the central tasks of deconstruction from the beginning: to refuse binary oppositions, particularly all of the forms of the opposition between nature and culture, including animal and man, and grown and made. In the discussion of cloning, interviewer Roudinesco expresses a concern that resonates with Habermas's views when she worries that certain ideas about cloning make human beings into machines (2004, 47). The machine occupies a special place in Derrida's thought. Indeed, the machine operates between nature and culture. We could say that machines haunt both (because there is never just one machine, but a multiplicity of machines). There are mechanistic and technical operations in both nature (or the grown) and in culture (or the made), which is just one of the reasons why this distinction is not fixed or absolute. Insofar as techniques and mechanisms are definitive of both sides of this binary, the two poles may not be as opposed as philosophers such as Harris and Habermas make them out to be.

Rather than worry that humans will become like machines, Derrida suggests that much of human experience is already mechanistic, and that we cannot be so sure that we are free while machines are not. Just as he refuses the opposition between man and animal, he refuses the opposition between man and machine. When we think of machines, we think of mechanistic determinism as opposed to human freedom. Yet for Derrida neither machines nor freedom can be reduced or defined in terms of a simple opposition. More importantly, he argues that we must not ignore or discount the machine, but instead must look for it everywhere. This is another aspect of deconstructive ethics, namely to vigilantly attempt to differentiate between response and reaction, or ethical decisions and mere moral rule-following; our attempts must be ongoing because we can never be sure, even in our "freest" moments or most intimate personal decisions, that we are not operating like machines, merely reacting rather than responding (see chapter 7). In addition, we should not underestimate machines, which may be more complex than we think (cf. Derrida 2004, 48). The opposition is not between human freedom (which, á la Habermas, will be compromised by genetic engineering and cloning) and the determinism of nature (which, á la Harris, we can seek to control or overcome through genetic engineering and cloning), since both nature and culture are machines of sorts.

The Excess in the Machine

Derrida defines the machine as "a system [dispositive] of calculation and repetition. As soon as there is calculation, calculability, and repetition, there is something of a machine. . . . But in the machine there is an excess in relation to the machine itself: at once the effect of a machination and something that eludes machinelike calculation" (2004, 49). And it is this excess in the machine that we could call freedom: "If freedom is an excess of play in the machine, an excess of every determinate machine, then I would militate for a recognition of and a respect for this freedom, but I prefer to avoid speaking of the subject's freedom or the freedom of man" (2004, 48). This excess or freedom, however, does not reside on just one side of the machine-human binary or the nature-culture binary, the human side, as some assume. Because the machine inhabits both, both are mechanistic. But this does not mean that they are determined in a fatalistic way. Derrida insists on excess and interruption within the operations of the machine itself. Rather, this excess appears as an interruption of the machine in nature and in culture, the encounter with the other, or what Derrida sometimes calls *the event*.[9]

The event cannot be calculated, predicted, mastered, or controlled. If it could be entirely predicted and controlled, it would be merely the mechanical operation of some machine or other. Again, this is not to say that there is such a thing as the machine or the mechanical *in itself*, the pure machine. On the other hand, if, as Harris imagines, genetic engineering could eliminate the "natural lottery of life," along with accident and chance, then everything could and would be calculable and controllable. This stance is untenable on the practical or empirical level, insofar as every individual being is unique, even if at the same time he or she (if sexual difference applies) inherits or repeats something of his or her ancestors, whoever they might be. Moreover, this view disrespects the otherness of the other, or what Derrida might call the *arrival* or *arrival-ness* of the other. It does not allow for surprises or radical differences that inhabit even what is most similar, even the clone. Furthermore, even while this view takes the side of the machine, so to speak, by embracing the idea that the future can be predicted and controlled, it also imagines us, the human engineers of that future, as somehow outside of the machine, the masters of it.

Again, in the context of discussing new technologies of cloning and machines, Derrida says:

> [A]n event worthy of the name can and ought to be, an *arrivance* that would surprise me absolutely and to whom or for whom, to which, or for which I could not, and may no longer, *not respond*—in a way that is as responsible as possible: what happens, what arrives and comes down upon me, that to which I am exposed, beyond all mastery. Heteronomy, then—the other is my law. What thus comes down on me does not necessarily come to me in order to elect me, as me, by presenting itself before me, in such a way that I *see it coming* horizontally, like an object or a subject that can be anticipated against the background of a horizon or a foreseeable future. There is no *horizon* for the other, any more than there is for death. (2004, 52)

Unlike for Habermas, however, the "threat" of otherness, even of the other-than-human, does not lead Derrida to oppose genetic engineering or cloning (although he does not unconditionally embrace them, either). Rather, Derrida maintains that in all relations with both "the grown and the made" there always have been forms of cloning. And all relations with others, whether they are grown or made, are "threatening" insofar as they challenge the authority and freedom of the sovereign subject, whether that subject is the scientist, the parent, or the child. Moreover, *contra* both Harris and Habermas, Derrida's remarks suggest that any response to others who may come, whether clones or otherwise, are inherently unforeseeable and beyond all mastery. In other words, whether children are "grown or made," they usher in a future that cannot be mastered by scientists, by parents, or by themselves. The freedom imagined by both Harris (rightfully on the side of the scientists and parents) and Habermas (rightfully on the side of the children) is always already "contaminated" by the machine.

This is why Derrida also insists that responsibility comes *before* freedom and not the reverse (2004, 52). We are not the autonomous sovereign agents assumed in debates over genetic engineering, yet we are responsible. And our supposed freedom does not follow from our capabilities, willful, rational, or otherwise. Indeed, ethics requires taking responsibility for that which we cannot foresee or predict, what we cannot will or know. More than this, it requires what Derrida calls a kind of "passive" decision that both acknowledges that what comes cannot be controlled or mastered, and takes responsibility for it anyway, even welcomes it, particularly in the case of the child. Our relation to the past and to the future is this sort of "double injunction" to receive and to choose by risking deciding in the face of what is undecidable (cf. 2004, 8). *Contra* Habermas, this "passive" decision in the face of the undecidable is not one that is within my abilities or determined by my sovereignty—otherwise it is not really a decision in the sense of response, but only a mechanical reaction. Echoing Kierkegaard, Derrida maintains that "between knowledge and decision a leap is required" (2004, 53), which means that although I may be obliged to gather as much knowledge as possible, since ultimately I cannot know for sure, I must risk deciding. More importantly, I must acknowledge the risk insofar as I give up my illusions of sovereignty and mastery, illusions that short-circuit ethical response.[10]

If we begin with the assumption of a sovereign agent who freely decides based on the "laws" of science or scientific knowledge, then we risk forgoing ethics for the sake of empty moral rules or principles. This is not a criticism of science. Rather, it is a criticism of the notion of freedom as mastery or sovereignty, a criticism that begins with a challenge to the opposition between freedom and determinism supposed in these debates, the opposition between the machine and the human. Derrida says: "Between the machinelike and the non-machinelike, then, there is a complex relation at work that is not a simple opposition. We can call it freedom, but only beginning at the moment when there is something incalculable. And I would also distinguish between an incalculable that remains homogeneous with calculation (and which escapes it for contingent reasons, such as finitude, a limited power, etc.) and a noncalculable that in essence would no longer belong to the order of calculation. The event—which in essence should remain unforeseeable and therefore not programmable—would be that which exceeds the machine. What would be necessary to try to think, and this is extremely difficult, is the event *with* the machine" (2004, 49).

Derrida's notion of the event with the machine presents a challenge to the approaches to genetic engineering of both Harris and Habermas. Whereas Harris thinks that the machine will give us mastery over the lottery of life, Derrida insists on the excess in the machine that makes the future beyond our control. And whereas Habermas worries about the disappearance of contingency necessary for moral decision making and the moral community, Derrida describes an ethical imperative beyond finite considerations of contingencies, which, while relevant, are merely symptoms of a more radical infinite otherness beyond reason and beyond communication.[11] Our responsibility to decide does not come merely from the contingencies of life or from the accidental—or from freedom from the machine of nature—but from excesses in the order of the machine itself. In other words, there is no pure machine. Rather, there is always interruption.[12] And the interruption of the event described by Derrida (what precisely cannot be described) is not just the result of contingencies of everyday life (including race and gender) that force us to decide to act this way or that way by negotiating between the demands of our bodies and the demands of our culture. Instead, Derrida is pointing to an ethical imperative beyond the moral community of sovereign, rational decision makers that obligates us to something beyond calculation, not because we do not know or cannot determine—because life is contingent—but rather because this other comes from an incalculable order that is in excess of our sovereignty. It is not because we do not know, but rather because we cannot know. It is not because we do not have the power that we might have or could have, but rather because we are powerless. This is what Habermas misses in the very Kierkegaard passage he cites to make his point about embracing or choosing one's lot in life. He misses that we not only are forced to choose, but also that we are responsible even for what we do not, and cannot, choose. Whereas Habermas's moral community is based on the sovereignty of the subject with finite moral duties agreed upon by rational agents, Derrida's hyperbolic ethics comes from the other beyond any subjective agency or sovereignty and brings with it infinite responsibility for both the accidental or contingent and the necessary or determined, as they are called.

Once the oppositional binaries *nature-culture, grown-made, determined-free* are deconstructed, ethical or moral principles lose any firm grounding in one side of the binary of the other. For if we can no longer appeal to something purely natural/grown or something purely technological/made, then we no longer have recourse to the very terms that set up the debate between philosophers such as Harris and Habermas. If there is always some technology at the heart of what we take to be natural (a claim Derrida makes throughout his work), and if there is always something of the machine in the cultural, then to prefer one over the other for its own sake no longer makes sense. This is especially problematic for Habermas, who argues against positive genetics on the grounds of human nature, or the grown, versus what is made via technology. But it is also problematic for Harris, who assumes that we can stand as sovereign agents outside of the machine of nature to control it. Derrida insists that human life—and all of life—operates between two machines, the machine of nature and the machine of culture (what in *The Beast and the Sovereign* he calls between two marionettes, as I discuss in chapter 3).

"As if Cloning Began with Cloning!"

Once we give up the fixed and absolute opposition between these two sides, or two machines, it becomes clear how Derrida can say that there has always been cloning. And we can see that his deconstructive project has, in some sense, always been about cloning. It is not far-fetched to say that his project has always been about reproduction, whether we are talking about the reproduction of humans or reproduction in art, literature, and philosophy. In his interview with Roudinesco, he says: "As if cloning began with cloning! As if there weren't cloning and then more cloning! As if there weren't a clonelike way of reproducing the discourse against cloning. . . . Wherever there is repetition and duplication, even resemblance, there is cloning—that is, wherever there is 'nature' and 'culture,' which are never without some kind of cloning" (2004, 38).[13] There has always been cloning in the sense that there has always been reproduction of the same; here Harris would agree with Derrida (see Harris 2004, 28). But this does not mean that the same is identical as opposed to different in a fixed binary like the other traditional oppositions that fuel these debates. Rather, Derrida introduces his concept of *différance* into the discussion of cloning in order to undermine the opposition between identity or sameness and difference or otherness, along with other oppositions, including that between human and machine.

As usual with his deconstructive strategy, Derrida prefers *both/and* to the *either/or* of traditional philosophy. With cloning, as with all reproduction, there is both sameness or identity and otherness or difference. Given that our language contributes to our categorizing of everything into one or the other, Derrida invents a new term to circumvent the tendency toward simple oppositions. He introduces *différance* early in his work.[14] For example, in *Of Grammatology*, he calls *différance* "[a]n economic concept designating the production of differing/deferring" (1976, 23). And he describes *différance* as what makes the opposition of presence and absence possible (1976, 143). In *Margins of Philosophy*, he explains that the Latin verb *differre* has two distinct meanings: to defer and to differ. And these two meanings suggest the operation of signification, which is to say, the operation of reproduction that plays between identity and difference, sameness and otherness (cf. 1982, 11).

In his discussion of cloning, Derrida applies the concept of *différance* to life and the reproduction of life. He explicates how this notion moves between identity and difference: "At certain 'moments,' this differance can interrupt these laws [natural or genetic laws]; at other moments, it can introduce the economy of a new configuration into the immanence of the living being. The interruption itself belongs to the field of what is genetically or biologically possible. These are not only different 'moments' of differance. Differance means at once *the same* (the living being, but deferred, relayed, replaced by a substitute supplement, by a prosthesis, by a supplementation in which 'technology' emerges) and *the other* (absolutely heterogeneous, radically different, irreducible and untranslatable, the aneconomic, the wholly-other or death). An interruption involving differance is both reinscribed into the economy of the same and opened to an excess of the wholly other" (2004, 40).

Even in the repetitions of the so-called laws of nature and the codes of genetics there are interruptions. There is otherness within sameness such that we are always other to ourselves in ways that interrupt or surprise and prevent any mastery of ourselves, let alone of others or generations to come, whether they are genetically engineered or not (a distinction that is also challenged by Derrida's deconstruction of the opposition between nature and culture and his insistence that there is always a technological supplement at the heart of what we take to be natural).

Derrida's hyperbolic ethics is based on an obligation that comes from the interruption of the other, an obligation to receive, to welcome it, even beyond one's own control or mastery. We have an obligation to welcome the future, not as fatalism, but as being infinitely responsible for it. Informed by Emmanuel Levinas, Derrida extends Kierkegaardian ethics and responsibility in a hyperbolic ethics that includes responsibility not only for one's own body and actions but also for others and for the Other, over whom and over which we have no control. We are not, as both Harris and Habermas maintain, the owners of our bodies. Neither are we sovereign agents who can control our own destinies or plan for human beings to come. Derrida's hyperbolic ethics insists on a radical responsibility in the face of the deconstruction of the sovereign unified subject, wherein our responsibility is not derived from our own free will or free choice. Rather, our responsibility comes from the Other and others to which and to whom we are beholden, others whom we do not even recognize. We are forced to decide between alternatives, to make ethical choices, even though we lack any absolute knowledge of good and evil. The irrational, nonmeaning, and accidental elements inherent in the contingencies of life not only force us to make rational decisions, to exercise our sovereignty to choose, as Habermas suggests. In addition, they undermine the very notion that we are sovereign, rational agents in a community based on rational communication. What if none of these are possible? What if we/humans do not possess the very capabilities upon which both Habermas and Harris found their different versions of liberalism? What happens to the possibility of the moral community? Moreover, what if the destruction of what Dworkin, and perhaps even Habermas, call morality and the moral community is necessary for any opening onto ethics? Only from the anxious space of undecidability is there a chance of making a "good" decision. For Derrida, we can avoid the worst only by taking responsibility for its possibility.

If morality becomes a matter of norms and conventions, then insofar as it provides a set of rules that allow for acting without the struggle of decision making, it is not ethical. An ethics that remains open to the other, to the unexpected and even unrecognized, requires giving up moral norms as universal rules of action. If doing good is a matter of rule or convention, then ethics is reduced to an unthinking allegiance to law, a learned reaction. Hyperbolic ethics insists on an infinite responsibility beyond morality insofar as morality is a matter of calculation and rules. Calculation, rules, and laws turn what should be an ethical response to the singularity of the other (or the event) into a mere reaction or reflex determined by convention. Derrida acknowledges that this challenge also calls into question the foundations of freedom and responsibility that traditionally ground ethics and morality. Yet he maintains that this constant questioning of foundations is essential to hyperbolic ethics: "On the one hand, casting doubt on responsibility, on decision, on one's own being-ethical, seems to me to be—and is perhaps what should forever remain—the unrescindable essence of ethics: decision and responsibility. Every firm knowledge, certainty, and assurance on this subject would suffice, precisely, to confirm the very thing one wishes to disavow, namely the reactionality in the response" (2003, 128). Derrida's early work on Rousseau in *Of Grammatology* (1976) demonstrates how the distinction between necessity and accident cannot hold up. There is an accident at the heart of the necessary, and therefore ethics is always without solid ground (cf. Oliver 2010).

Derrida's hyperbolic ethics cautions us not to draw the line between right and wrong, good and evil, or healthy and unhealthy in a fixed or rigid way; to do so is not only to become reactionary rather than responsive, but also, and moreover, to shirk an ethical responsibility to the radical openness and fluidity of all moral categories. In this sense, ethics provides a kind of corrective for morality. If morality divides the world into good and evil, then hyperbolic ethics demands that we constantly question that division and our own investment in it.

In conclusion, mainstream debates over genetic enhancement and cloning not only assume a clear-cut opposition between nature as determined and humanity as free sovereign agents, but also assume that through genetic engineering we can master the accidental or contingent elements of existence through tinkering with genetic code. Some, like Harris, argue for this, while others, like Habermas, argue against it. Certainly, if the misplaced arrogance of medical science has taught us anything, it is that even in the best of circumstances, we cannot control life, which is full of accidents and surprises. The imagined control over reproduction suggested in these debates seems far from actual practices that still require implantation in women's wombs and all of the uncontrollable and unexpected consequences that follow, not to mention the unpredictability of genetic combinations and the profound influence of nurture on the resulting children. Some philosophers such as Harris are reassured that genetic engineering can eliminate these contingencies from reproduction, while others such as Dworkin and Habermas argue that contingencies are necessary for moral decision-making and responsibility, suggesting perhaps that we choose our children precisely because we cannot control them. For these philosophers, however, our responsibility follows from the certainty of our own authorship of our decisions and actions in the face of the contingencies of life. In either case, these philosophers stake their claims on the sovereign freedom of human will and the authorship of its decisions.

Both John Harris's moral imperative to enhance and Jürgen Habermas's species ethics disavow the ambiguities of life. Only by embracing ambiguity— or at least acknowledging that we cannot master it—can we hope to avoid the violence that results from the abjection of ambiguity in favor of neat categories that exclude the messiness of life. If we start from these ambiguities and ground an ethics there, rather than on abstract moral norms or some notion of humanity as a species, then our ethics comes out of, instead of against, the contingencies of life as we actually live it. As we learn from Derrida's hyperbolic ethics, our responsibility is no less because we cannot control those contingencies or because we are not masters of ourselves or of others. Rather, our responsibility is the result of a call from the other/Other who/that does not meet our expectations and does not fall neatly into one category or another. Ethics begins where moral rules leave off, in the realm of the undecidable, where the ambiguities of life abound and we are powerless in the face of them. Ethics begins with the "passive" decision to welcome otherness, even—perhaps especially—others that may threaten our sense of ourselves as sovereign masters of our own destinies.

Again, in the context of discussing cloning, Derrida says: "[Hospitality] may well be one of the names for what is in question here: to welcome, in an inventive way—with some genuine effort and good will—the one who or which comes into one's home, and comes to oneself, inevitably, without invitation. . . . Pure or unconditional hospitality assumes that the one arriving has not been invited to the place where I remain master of my domain and where I control my house, my territory, my language, where (according, on the contrary, to rules of conditional hospitality) he should in some way conform to the accepted rules of the place that welcomes him. Pure hospitality consists in leaving one's house open to the unforeseeable arrival, which can be an intrusion, even a dangerous intrusion, liable eventually to cause harm" (2004, 59). Genetic engineering brings with it unforeseeable arrivals, even intrusions. But these surprises are not unique to technology; rather, cloning has been here all along in sexual reproduction and all forms of the reproduction of life with its repetitions of sameness combined with the singularity of each living being. This ambiguity of the both/and may threaten the fixed categories that give us a sense of security; but only by accepting and embracing this ambiguity can we begin to welcome the happening of life. In a sense, we are all like Caster Semenya, both/and rather than either/or. Because "nature is a slob," in order to live together we need to learn to accept, if not enjoy, the mess.

TWO

Artificial Insemination: Deconstructing *Choice* versus *Chance*

> *Does one invent a child?* If the child invents himself, is it as the specular
> invention of parental narcissism or is it as the other who, in speaking and
> responding, becomes the absolute invention, the irreducible transcendent
> of what is nearest, all the more heterogeneous and inventive in that it
> seems to respond to parental desire? The truth of the child, therefore,
> would invent itself in a sense that would be neither that of unveiling nor
> that of discovery, neither that of creation nor that of production. It would
> be found where truth is thought beyond any inheritance.
>
> —JACQUES DERRIDA, *Psyche: Invention of the Other*
>   (emphasis added)

In an age when a child could have as few as one or as many as three genetic
parents, maternity and paternity have become tricky business. For example,
only one "parent" is necessary for cloning, while current experiments
make it possible to combine nuclear DNA from one woman, mitochondrial
DNA from another woman, and DNA from a man's sperm, which makes
three genetic parents. Add the contributions from a gestational carrier,
who could be a third woman, and the child has four parents to whom he or
she is biologically indebted, if not also genetically related; and then add still
different parents who raise the child, the so-called social parents, and even in
a traditional two-parent household, as many as six parents could be contributing to the genetic, biological, and social parenting of a child. But assisted
reproduction not only has made maternity and paternity tricky business,
but also has made it big business, indeed a billion-dollar industry.
Reproduction as business, and so-called designer babies, raise the question

of the relationship between parents and patents. Can parents *design* their babies? Can they not only intentionally choose to reproduce, but also choose what kind of baby to conceive? With cloning and genetic engineering, can parents invent their children? Can certain genetic traits be patented? Are parents becoming patents? Reproduction has become a form of production where genetic materials are bought and sold as the raw materials with which to make a baby. Certainly, the fact that sperm donors, egg donors, and surrogates are paid for biological materials and labor makes some people—especially the children conceived through such technologies—uneasy about making babies into sales transactions (see Marquardt 2010).[1]

These technological advances in reproduction lead to new legal problems in how to define a family. Who counts as a mother or a father when genetic or biological material from several adults is used (egg donor, sperm donor, gestational carrier)?[2] Until the advent of paternity tests, fatherhood was a matter of testimony (from women and men). Maternity, however, has traditionally been considered obvious. But with technologies that make it possible to have three women contribute biologically to the conception and gestation of the child, and the possibility that another—or other—women may raise him or her, the question of who is the mother becomes even more problematic than the question of who is the father.[3] Imagine, for example, an ovum created from the eggs of two women, which is then inseminated, and the fertilized egg implanted in a third woman who acts as gestational carrier for two women, say a lesbian couple, who plan to raise the child as their own: Do we have one mother, two mothers, or five?

Although using eggs from two women is only in experimental stages and is being considered for the prevention of certain diseases, using egg donors and gestational carriers is becoming more common every year. Three "mothers" is not so unusual. In fact, many infertile women who use surrogates or gestational carriers prefer that their child be conceived using donor eggs, so that the baby will not be genetically related to the carrier; the rationale is that if the child is not genetically related to her, the carrier will be less likely to sue for custody. These reproductive realities have created complicated legal problems in defining mothers and parents. Traditionally, the mother is the woman who gives birth to the child. But with the increase in the number of cases of what used to be called *surrogate mothers*, now called *gestational carriers*—a telling shift in itself—the woman who gives birth to a child is no longer necessarily considered its mother (we cannot refer to the woman who gives birth as the *birth mother*, because that is a technical term that refers to a woman who gives her child up for adoption). Using the term *mother* has become difficult. And even the law is decidedly ambiguous with regard to who is considered a mother. In the words of Elizabeth Marquardt, "When the woman carrying the embryo not conceived with her own egg intends to be the mother, we call her the 'mother' and the other woman the 'egg donor.' But when the woman who gives the egg intends to be the mother, we call *her* the 'mother' and the woman carrying the embryo conceived with that egg the 'gestational surrogate.'. . . Either way, the result is an embryo and—ultimately—a child conceived from one woman's egg, fertilized by the sperm of a man (who we call either the 'father' or the 'sperm donor'), and carried in another woman's womb" (Marquardt, 2011, 45).

Certainly, these transactions are legally complicated in that they are usually handled through contracts that are *more or less* legally binding and involve payment for genetic material, sperm or eggs, and gestational labor, including childbirth. They are business deals. And the so-called intentional parents can select what "kind" of sperm or egg they want, and to some extent who they want to carry their child (although this task is usually only taken up by women who need money).

Derrida's question, "Does one invent the child?" takes on a literal hue in light of today's reproductive technologies. In 1984 when Derrida asked this question, however, using egg donors was not yet possible, and surrogacy was virtually unheard of (until the next year, when Mary Beth Whitehead sued for custody of "Baby M," conceived with her own egg and the sperm of William Stern, who contracted with her to have a baby that he and his wife would then adopt). Although Derrida's primary concern was with a paradox in the concept of invention and not literally with inventing children, his analysis is uncanny given recent developments in reproductive technology and the conceptual difficulties that ensue. Derrida's discussion is motivated by a more general wonder about the possibility of inventing something new, something other; yet his deconstruction of the oppositions between discovery and creation (what in the last chapter we called *grown* and *made*), legitimate and illegitimate, original and copy, heir and bastard, are startlingly relevant to current discussions around questions of reproduction.[4]

In part, Derrida traces a genealogy of the concept of invention from the idea that invention is *finding* something new that no one had seen before, to invention as *creating ex nihilo*, and contemporary issues of patents, patent law, and ownership. Derrida argues that as the notion of invention transforms from discovery to ownership, so too the role of chance or luck is transformed into necessity, as the genius inventor claims the right to ownership of his ideas and the products of them. As we will see, this transition from luck or chance to choice and ownership applies to current debates around genetic engineering and "designer babies," and the changing relationship between parents and patents.

In light of new reproductive technologies, especially certain forms of assisted reproductive technologies (ARTs) that use donor eggs and/or sperm, genetic engineering, and the possibility of cloning, the question "Does one invent the child?" takes on a new meaning, particularly in terms of the discourse of sovereign ownership. With ARTs, becoming a parent seems a matter of design in ways that were not possible until recently, which raises this question anew and requires us to rethink—if not reinvent—the meaning of parenthood, kinship, genealogy, and inheritance. Derrida's analysis of inheritance in terms of *traditio* as tradition, transfer, and translation is relevant here as inheritance becomes a matter of genetic transfer, and parentage becomes a matter of legal interpretation. So-called designer babies and the idea that we can invent our own children through genetic engineering and cloning make Derrida's analysis of invention all the more pressing. These technologies through which we intervene in human reproduction compel us to reconsider long-held oppositions between nature and technology, nature and culture, real and artificial, and given and made. The deconstruction of these oppositions comes into play in a new field, one in which the very terms of the debate may change as a result.

Indeed, as we have seen, within current debates in bioethics, new reproductive technologies—particularly genetic engineering and cloning—are framed between the two poles of nature and culture, with proponents falling out on the side of culture or technology (or the made) and detractors on the side of nature (or the given). Many of these discussions revolve around some sense of *real* versus *artificial* reproduction, and *natural* versus *man-made* human offspring. Of interest to me is the way in which these current debates resuscitate the ancient triangulation between technology (*techne*), nature (*physis*), and chance (*tyche*), which seems to have been lost to philosophical articulations of the relation between nature and technology at least since the dualism of seventeenth-century modern philosophy and Romantic philosophies of nature of the eighteenth century. Yet some discourses return us to this triad precisely by disavowing the role of chance in invention and assuming that technology gives us control over our destiny as human beings. This is what bioethicist John Harris calls replacing the "natural lottery" of nature and the randomness of natural evolution with the "mastery" of human reproduction and evolution "enhanced" through technological control.

Derrida's deconstruction of the opposition between nature and culture, especially as he applies it explicitly to the problem of surrogacy, provides an important counterpoint to current debates in bioethics. For, well before recent advances in ARTs, genetic engineering, and cloning, Derrida revealed the connection between mother and nature as a fable that covers over both technology and chance, which are always already at the origin of humanity. Decades ago, Derrida was already asking, "Who is the mother?" Here, I use what Derrida calls *deconstructive genealogy* in order to unsettle the opposition between nature and culture that continues into debates over new reproductive technologies. What I hope to insert into these debates over assisted reproduction is the inescapability of chance on both sides of the nature-technology divide, especially as that opposition plays itself out in current discussions of assisted reproductive technologies.

The Mother-Effect

In the beginning of *Psyche: Inventions of the Other*, Derrida calls the paradox of invention "the *question of the son*," teasing and yet somehow reassuring his reader that "this question happens also to be a scene of *traditio* as tradition, transfer, and translation; we could also say it is an allegory or metaphor" (1984, 4). He signals that although he is going to call into question the "question of the son," the legitimate heir, at the same time this question is metaphorical.[5] Figures of legitimate and bastard sons haunt much of Derrida's work (cf. Krell 2000). Indeed, one way to interpret Derrida's overall project from his earliest texts to his last—a questionable gesture to say the least, especially when legitimacy and translation are always at stake there—is as an attempt to demonstrate how what we take to be legitimate or proper sons or heirs are really, if truth be told, bastards. At one level, this is why he links truth to testimony and secret in his later work; after all, paternity, and more especially legitimacy, traditionally have been a matter of a father's testimony—or his secret. And now new reproductive technologies, especially egg donors and gestational carriers, make motherhood a matter of testimony too. Just as the father was once considered to be whoever claimed to be the father, the mother is whoever claims to be the mother.

Throughout his work, Derrida suggests that behind the question of the legitimate or proper son is the question of the illegitimate or improper mother.[6] He shows us that the mother remains the hidden secret that secures legitimacy, even as an identification with her threatens to upset patriarchy. Derrida works his "deconstructive genealogy" on figures throughout the history of philosophy and literature to demonstrate that behind their claims of propriety, truth, and transparency, or behind their claims of genius, creativity, and self-birth, is the fantasy of a maternal origin that remains hidden, disavowed, or buried; and their claims to a proper place in intellectual history are based upon this *improper* relation with a dead mother, with a matricide they have committed in order to keep her close.[7] Behind all claims to propriety, property, and what is "proper to man" lies an animal-mother-God whose existence is both presupposed and hidden. She remains outside of the law and therefore her son can inhabit it, even transgress it. In other words, the son claims his legitimate place by fetishizing a maternal origin, which is to say simultaneously idealizing it and disavowing it in an attempt to give birth to himself without her. This Dr. Frankenstein approach to creating human life without sex and without women continues to be one of the fantasies operating in debates over genetic engineering, cloning, and new reproductive technologies generally, as imagined by predominantly male bioethicists.

Of course, the mother and her various surrogates are at the very beginnings of Derrida's deconstructive project. Jean-Jacques Rousseau's absent/ dead mother is a central figure in Derrida's now-classic *Of Grammatology* (1976). There, Derrida argues that in Rousseau's texts the myth of an original mother, of mother-nature, is produced through a chain of supplements or replicas of her, which in turn "produce the sense of the very thing they defer" (1976, 157). He maintains that "the absolute present, Nature, that which words like 'real mother' name, have always already escaped, have never existed" (1976, 159). The *mother-effect*, as we might call it, is the result of the absence of a real mother, who is therefore mythologized and romanticized as the origin and plentitude of Nature, but whose disappearance is a prerequisite for the myth itself. Echoing yet parodying Rousseau, Derrida concludes, "the displacing of the relationship with the mother, with nature, with being as the fundamental signified, such indeed is the origin of society and languages" (1976, 266).[8] Operating within the binaries *nature-culture* and *life-death*, which he associates with several proper names in the history of philosophy, including Rousseau, Derrida "deconstructs" them by showing how what is taken to be original—nature, or life—is already contaminated by culture, or death.[9] As we will see, Derrida's deconstruction of origin, originals, along with the original of mother-nature, have significant implications for discussions of surrogacy, cloning, and other reproductive technologies that make it increasingly difficult to identify the mother or the original.

Once Derrida points it out in *Of Grammatology*, this play of substitute mothers becomes obvious in Rousseau's texts, starting with Rousseau's confession of his first love, Madame de Warens, whom he called *Mamma*, through his love for Thérèse, whom he called "the substitute [*supplément*] that I needed" (1976, 156–57). Rousseau's "real" mother died in childbirth, and the story of his life is populated with substitutes for this missing mother. Moreover, his philosophy postulates an original Mother Nature, perfect in herself, who is corrupted by man's evil and human culture (cf. 1976, 145). Derrida traces this fable of original (maternal) plenitude and perfection throughout the history of philosophy in order to show how lack and corruption are not only already present at its heart, but also how they are necessary to create the mother-effect. Thus, there is a substitute or surrogate mother already in the place of the original. Mother Nature is an invention, a fable, created through the matricidal movements of a philosophy claiming to give birth to itself, to invent itself.

The Fable of Invention, or the Luck of the Draw

Whereas *invention* once meant to find something for the first time, something already there, it has come to mean to create something new, something that can be patented and thereby owned, controlled, and distributed (cf. Derrida 2007a, 29–30). Invention has become property in an economy of the proper, not only in terms of material resources owned but also in terms of capacities possessed, namely, the capacity to create and control, to bring into being. Invention/creation, then, becomes the truth of man, that he creates and controls things, beings, substances, devices and so forth that can be patented. In other words, he invents himself as the self-reproducing creator *ex nihilo* of the truth about himself and his proper place in the world. Throughout his work, Derrida maintains that this illusion of control and mastery, of the proper place of man—the legitimate son—operates according to a logic of the supplementary, whereby man claims originality, creativity, even genius by reproducing himself as the agent or master of production/reproduction while assuming the plenitude of a nature he both denies and covets (cf. 2007a, 43).

Thus, man always and only invents himself and never anything other: "Invention comes down or back to the same, and this is always possible, as soon as it can receive a status and thereby be legitimatized by an institution that it then becomes in its turn. For what is being invented in this way are always institutions. Institutions are always inventions and the inventions to which a status is conferred are in turn institutions" (2007a, 43). Insofar as the "invention" is named and patented as legitimate and proper, it is institutionalized in a way that recuperates it into the economy of the same, and often literally into the economy of capital where it can be owned, bought, and sold. (As Heidegger might say, it becomes standing reserve, and so do we, insofar as we think that we can create/own ourselves.) As we will see, this is becoming the case with ARTs and genetic engineering that produce "designer babies" and clones, wherein, if our science fiction is any indication, the clone is imagined as a product rather than a person. Some scientists, some members of the medical establishment, and some bioethicists describe reproductive technologies in terms of invention, ownership, and patents. *Parents are becoming patents* such that certain genes are worthy of reproducing and others are not. (Think of the sci-fi films *Moon* and *The Island*, for example.) And we begin to imagine that we can control our own DNA, our own evolution, making parents into patents for "enhancing evolution" and making "better people," as bioethicist John Harris says. This scenario evokes science-fiction dystopias such as that imaged in the film *Gattaca*, where the genetically enhanced dominate those who haven't been enhanced.

"Designer Babies" or "Accidental Pregnancies"?

The myth that man gives birth to himself through his inventiveness becomes the myth that man has the capacity to create himself, even to create life itself—myth become reality through technologies of genetic engineering and cloning. Yet in a sense man's inventiveness or capacity to create—to create even himself—is produced through a fable in which man is the protagonist and hero. This fable of mastery and invention applies to the dominant narratives of, and debates over, genetic engineering and cloning, premised as they are on whether or not we should control our own repro-duction, or "play God." This assumes, of course, that the science of repro-duction and technologies of reproduction offer such mastery—and therein lies the fable. A deconstructive genealogy of invention reveals the place (and disavowal) of chance and luck, which is missing from the narrative of genetic mastery through science and technology.

Again, Derrida's conceptual analysis of parents versus patents in fables of invention applies full force to questions of genetic engineering and cloning, as well as to reproductive technologies that make it possible to buy biologi-cal material and the rights to use it to conceive babies "by design." As Derrida suggests, in order for man to take himself as the author and agent of his own creations, he must discount the role of chance, luck, and even discovery; he doesn't discover what is there, see it for the first time already there before him, but invents it, creates it, possesses it as his own. His sense of himself as maker, as *homo faber*, is dependent upon the separation of tech-nology and chance. Speaking of Leibniz, Derrida says:

> The role of inventor (a genius or ingenious) is precisely to have that chance—
> and, in order to do so, not to fall upon the truth by chance, but, as it were,
> *to know chance, to know how to be lucky*, to recognize the luck of chance, to
> anticipate a chance, to decipher it, grasp it, inscribe it on the charter or the
> necessity and turn a throw of the dice into work. This transfiguration, which
> both preserves and nullifies chance as such, goes so far as to affect the very
> status of the aleatory event. (2007a, 38–39)

It is no accident (so to speak) that Derrida associates this throw of the dice at the heart of invention with dissemination, specifically in terms of the Stoics Epicurus and Lucretius and their notion of "seminal multiplicity," or the dissemination of the seed of things that allows for diversity in nature, that is, the Stoics' *logoi spermatikoi*, or seminal reasons. Speaking of the Stoics, Derrida concludes: "This theory of literal dissemination is also a discourse on incidents and accidents *as* symptoms. . . . [T]he sense of the fall in general (symptom, lapsus, incident, accidentality, cadence, coincidence, expiration date, luck, good luck, bad luck or *méchance*) is thinkable solely in the situation, the places, or space of finitude, within the multiple relation to the multiplicity of elements, letters, or seeds" (2007a, 351–52; note that *méchance* is a play on words, since the title of the essay from which the passage is quoted is "My Chances/*Mes chances*," and *méchanceté* also means cruelty/meanness/unkindness). That is, the logos or ordering principle of the *logoi spermatikoi* is possible only because of the dissemination of spermatikoi and its disordering effect. Whether or not the seed takes, and what comes of it if it does, is always a matter of chance and luck, and sometimes even of cruelty.

Freud's Accident

Derrida argues that certain strains in philosophy and psychoanalysis (and we might add contemporary bioethics, if not also science) have "reappropriat[ed] chance as necessity or inevitableness" (2007a, 374). Discussing Freud, Derrida maintains that the father of psychoanalysis eliminated chances and randomness in order to ground psychoanalysis as a proper science. He quotes a passage from "Leonardo da Vinci and a Memory of His Childhood" in which Freud seemingly contradicts his earlier claims that psychoanalysis has nothing to do with the chance accidents of Leonardo's birth: "[E]verything to do with our life is chance [*Zufall*], from our origin of the meeting of spermatozoon and ovum onwards [this is *also* what I call, in my language, dissemination]—chance which nevertheless has a share in the law and necessity of nature, and which merely lacks any connection with our wishes and illusions" (2007a, 376; brackets and italics are Derrida's). Derrida interprets the psychoanalytic impulse to find the cause of every symptom, the original trauma, the analytic meaning as itself a symptom, even an obsession.[10] Freudian psychoanalysis turns on interpreting what otherwise might be seen as accidents or symptoms in a scientific and deterministic logic of cause and effect. (It is noteworthy that the Greek *symptoma* also means *accident*.)

There may be, as Freud says, many causes in nature that we can never know, that lack any connection to our wishes or explanations; but Freud stakes his project on a distinction between natural causes, which may be a matter of chance (such as "accidents" of birth) and psychic causes, which can be interpreted, known, even cured. We might say that Freud is ambivalent toward nature, specifically toward Mother Nature, whom he associates with both life and death. He wants psychoanalysis to be taken seriously as a science, and yet he must distinguish it from the other sciences. (As I have argued elsewhere, Freud has an ambivalent relationship to science, which appears in his texts as a kind of science envy; see Oliver 1995 and 2009.) For his part, after demonstrating how Freud separates psychoanalysis from the natural sciences in order to argue that it is more scientific insofar as it is less accidental, Derrida concludes, "Freud loves nature and takes good care of it" (2007a, 376).

Given Derrida's analysis, we should add *Mother Nature*, because his deconstruction of the Freudian project on the double role of symptom—as the necessary effect of a discernable cause, on the one hand, and as a matter of chance or luck, on the other—revolves around a story of an old woman whom Derrida imagines as Freud's mother. In order to distinguish accidental or chance happenings from the proper purview of psychoanalytic interpretation or symptoms, Freud tells the story of his coachman taking him to the wrong address when he was making a house call to administer a shot of morphine and some eye drops to an elderly woman patient. Freud was so flustered when he arrived at the proper destination (after telling the coachman that he had made a wrong turn) that he dropped the morphine in the eye instead of giving it as a shot. Luckily, Freud says, it did no harm. With this story, he distinguishes between his mistake and the coachman's mistake. Whereas Freud's mistake has a cause in his unconscious that can be interpreted, his coachman's arriving at the wrong destination was an accident or chance that does not have further meaning for him and could not be relevant to his own psyche or his relationship to this patient, unless, as he says, he were superstitious, which he isn't, and saw it as an omen, since that year the old lady died (cf. Derrida 2007a, 366).

Reading this, Derrida begins to wonder if this old woman is really Freud's mother, and upon going back to the text discovers that although she cannot be his real mother, she represents Freud's mother and his fear of his mother's death (2007a, 368). I cannot recount all of the subtleties of Derrida's analysis here, but suffice it to say that he concludes by suggesting that despite Freud's attestations to the contrary, the good doctor could be mistaken in his interpretation, perhaps even in the entire enterprise of psychoanalysis, insofar as it claims the status of a science of discernable causes and effects, especially because those effects are always symptoms or accidents. He says, "Freud can still be mistaken about the address or the pharmakon, he can replace the eye drops with morphine, the old woman could be his mother or his mother-in-law, and the 'I' of the coachman is perhaps not an other. He is perhaps not good. Perhaps he is a bastard" (2007a, 376). He is perhaps not the good and legitimate son, and psychoanalysis is perhaps not the heir to legitimate science. For, under Derrida's deconstructive gaze, there is matricide behind this good son, just as it is behind so many others good sons from the history of philosophy. Behind every legitimate heir there is the possibility of their illegitimacy, the possibility that they are matricidal "bastards" who cannot be sure that their genealogy is not contaminated by the very principle, superstition, or uncertainty they wish to exclude.

Surrogacy, or the Fable of Genealogy

In Derrida's little-known essay "Who Is the Mother? Birth, Nature, Nation," and in an interview with Elizabeth Roudinesco in *For What Tomorrow*, he addresses the question of surrogacy head on, or "frontally," as he might say (1993b, 2004). If in his other work he has repeatedly reminded us of a metaphorical link in the history of philosophy and psychoanalysis between the insistence on certainty and maternity, here he makes the link literal. And I should quickly add that by so doing, he calls into question any certainty about the very distinction between the metaphorical and the literal or surrogate and real mothers. Continuing what he calls *deconstructive genealogy*, Derrida puts in question the traditional assumption that a child's mother is known with certainty since she carries and gives birth to the child (1993b). The mother has been taken to be a credible, even infallible, witness who is not only present at the child's birth, but also can testify beyond doubt to the child's parentage, to its genealogy. In addition, usually there are other witnesses to this mother's status as present at birth, even institutional ones like doctors, nurses, and other hospital staff, who, based on her testimony, sign official documents naming the mother, the father, and the child.

Until relatively recently, with the advent of paternity tests, however, paternity was inconclusive, sometimes incredible, except for testimony of a different sort, the testimony not of eyewitnesses but of expert witnesses, who testified to what cannot be seen. Traditionally, then, paternity has been based not on presence at the birth of the child, but rather on the word of one or both parents. And legitimacy was conferred on the child only when a man accepted paternal responsibility and named the child as his own. It is significant, however, that both mother and father gave their word, or testified, to something (conception) that no one actually witnesses; even if someone were to witness the sex, they would not witness the conception. For even now, when scientists can view or record images of the sperm penetrating the ovum, it is unclear whether or not they are witnessing conception. In most cases outside of laboratories, if the parents are present—and even here we might question what it means to be present— during the sexual act that leads to conception, we would not say that they are present at conception, even if we can define conception as sperm inseminating an egg, for (usually) no one *sees* that happen; there are no eyewitnesses. Indeed, what would it mean to say that anyone is present for, or to, that event? In most cases, it happens without anyone's knowledge or awareness.

In the past, paternity was sometimes the claim of a woman, the mother, against a man, named as the father. It was often a disputed claim, with opposing testimony from both sides and/or secret arrangements. Legitimacy was contingent upon the father admitting or accepting paternity and testifying to it. In other words, until the advent of paternity tests, legitimacy was the result of a man claiming fatherhood and giving a child his name. Without his testimony, the child would be considered illegitimate or a "bastard." Sperm donors further complicate paternity; legally, they are not considered fathers, yet they are biological fathers, possibly to numerous unknown offspring. With new reproductive technologies, motherhood too becomes a matter of testimony and witness, or speculation and secrets. Indeed, most women who use donor eggs to conceive do not tell their children—or anyone else—that they are not the "biological mothers" of their children, assuming of course that in this context the term *biological mother* still makes any sense (see Mundy 2007). And married women who use sperm donors usually look for donors with physical characteristics similar to their husbands' so that their children will "pass" as the biological offspring of both parents (see Quiroga 2007).

It is noteworthy that the first cases of artificial insemination were clandestine procedures in doctors' offices, where even the women involved didn't know the truth about their childrens' paternity. Reportedly, some doctors "helped" women conceive by anesthetizing them, inseminating them with their own sperm or the sperm of medical students, and then instructing the women to go home and have sex with their husbands that night. This was a "treatment" for cases of the husband's infertility, without either partner knowing of it or suspecting that the husband was not the biological father of the child. In other cases, the women were knowing participants, instructed not to tell anyone (see Marquardt 2010, 17). From such stories of late-nineteenth-century and early-twentieth-century donor insemination through to the present, donor-conceived children usually do not know that their "social father" is not their "biological father" (see Marquardt 2010, 17). Like all of us, they know only what their parents tell them, or what they find out from other relatives, or by accident.

If pregnancy and childbirth, and inheritance and illegitimacy, have always been matters of testimony and secrecy (at least since the nineteenth century, as evidenced by popular novels by authors such as Charles Dickens wherein the plot is often driven by an orphan's discovery of his or her inheritance or secret birthright), then new reproductive technologies provide another twist in possible secrets of birth. Certainly, new technologies have spawned all sorts of fantasies of birth involving secrets, testimony, and fantasies of origin. For example, the 2010 film *The Kids Are All Right* is the story of two children, conceived by their lesbian mothers through assisted reproduction involving a sperm donor, who go looking for their "biological father," the anonymous donor (see Oliver 2012). And children looking for their sperm-donor father are an ever-increasing internet presence. In addition to curiosity about biological fathers and fantasies of origins, some of these children are also driven by fears of "accidental incest" (Marquardt 2010). Since until recently there were very few regulations on sperm donation, one sperm donor could be biologically related to hundreds of children. Some worry about these sibling children becoming lovers and possibly producing their own offspring. Although it is not possible for an egg donor to donate as many eggs as one sperm donor can donate sperm, with the growing business of egg donation, secrets, longing for origins, and worries about accidental incest can haunt questions of maternity as well as questions of paternity.

The Mother as Legal Fiction

In "Who Is the Mother?" Derrida argues that "the mother was never less of a legal fiction than the father" (1993b). Certainly, new technologies have necessitated legal intervention into what was once considered natural, even obvious. Who counts as "the mother" is now a matter of legal definition in a way that it wasn't just decades ago. States are racing to keep up with new technologies that are making new family configurations possible, configurations with several mothers or fathers. When Derrida asked "who is the mother?" in 1993, egg donation was not yet a possibility. And although he discusses the impact of surrogacy on our conceptions of motherhood and family, his point is that these new technologies only highlight what has always been the case.

Derrida argues that "the original *physis* was always foreshadowed by *techne*, by the possibility of *techne*, that is the repeatability and replaceability, and haunted it with nightmarish force" (1993b). In this essay, he again calls on Freud to challenge the certainty of the mother and the uncertainty of the father that sets in motion representation and civil society. Discussing Freud's account of the Rat Man's obsessional neurosis, Derrida finds doubt at the heart of certainty, this time a certainty grounded in maternity. Derrida's analysis revolves around a footnote in which Freud quotes Lichtenberg saying, "An astronomer knows whether the moon is inhabited or not with about as much certainty as he knows who was his father, but not with so much certainty as he knows who was his mother." The lesson Freud draws from this comparison is that civilization made a "great advance" when representation replaced sense-certainty (in the form of patriarchy replacing matriarchy) with the need to witness or testify to something as a form of begetting (*Zeuge* in German means both *witness* and *begetter*; see Derrida 1993b; cf. 2004, 40). In other words, maternal certainty, which supposedly keeps us at the level of sense-certainty, is replaced by paternal uncertainty, which supposedly moves us to the level of representation, which is why Freud concludes the footnote by remarking that "in hieroglyphics the word for 'witness' is written with a representation of the male organ" (see Derrida 1993b). Insofar as paternity supposedly moves us away from our senses and the natural world and into representation and the cultural, it is seen as progress.

Derrida challenges this supposed certainty of maternal perception versus paternal judgment, suggesting not only that new technologies make it far from certain who is the mother, but also that we have never known—and can never know—our maternal (or paternal) origins with absolute certainty. Commenting on Freud's footnote on Lichtenberg, Derrida says:

> But this schema, even and especially in Freud, seems more fragile than ever. Today less than ever can we be sure that the mother herself is the woman we believe we saw giving birth. The mother is not only the genetrix since, as psychoanalysis (and not only psychoanalysis) has always taught us, another person can become or can have been "the" mother, one of the mothers. . . . In other words, the identity of the mother (like her possible juridical identification) depends on a judgment that is just as derived, and on an inference that is just as divorced from all immediate perception, as this "legal fiction" of a paternity conjectured through reason. (2004, 41)

The possibility of several women and several men being the mother(s) or father(s) is "accelerated" with new genetic technologies. But it has always been a possibility, indeed perhaps a characteristic of the human psyche that it takes, makes, and needs substitute mothers and substitute fathers, even if this means mothering or fathering itself. If psychoanalysis teaches us no other lesson, it is this one.

Derrida repeats this line of thought in "La Veilleuse," where he deconstructs what Jacques Trilling proposes as an "ontological distinction" between the mother and maternity, one natural and the other cultural. Derrida argues that like paternity, maternity has always also been a "legal fiction" (to use a phrase from James Joyce; see 2001b, 27). Here again he cites the Freudian footnote in order to call into question the certainty of the mother and of maternity, and to unseat the privilege given to paternity as testimony and representation and the denigration of maternity to mere sense-certainty (26). On this view, the mother is irreplaceable while the father can use, and is a matter of, substitution or symbols. He is the legal fiction, while she is the real *thing*. Extending his analysis to Lacan and Trilling, Derrida argues that the notion of the phallic mother changes nothing in this regard (27). The mother, like the father, is a phantasm, a fiction, always substitutable, always already a supplement for an absent fantastic origin: "the mother is also a speculative object and herself a legal fiction" (28; translation mine).

Commenting on "La Veilleuse," Michael Naas concludes, "In an age of frozen embryos, in vitro fertilization, and surrogate motherhood, we must today acknowledge, argues Derrida, what has in fact always been the case: the mother, like the father, is subject to 'substitution, rational inference, phantasmatic or symbolic construction, speculation, and so on'. In a word, the mother, like the father, is a legal fiction that risks becoming a sovereign phantasm, a legitimate or legitimated phantasm and a phantasm of legitimation. . . . Subject to phantasm, then, the mother is not natural but inscribed in history, in conventions, subject to symbolization, speculation, and replacement" (Naas 2008, 210). Naas quotes a passage from Derrida that I replicate here to show that the virtually unknown Hungarian lecture "Who Is the Mother?" is not unique in the Derridean corpus:

> If today the unicity of the mother is no longer the sensible object of a perceptual certitude, if maternities can no longer be reduced to, indeed if they carry us beyond, the carrying mother, if there can be, in a word, more than one mother, if "the" mother is the object of calculation and supposition, of projection and phantasm, if the "womb" is no longer outside all phantasm, the assured place of birth, this "new" situation simply illuminates in return an ageless truth. The mother was never only, never uniquely, never indubitably the one who gives birth—and whom one sees, with one's own eyes, give birth. (quoted in Naas 2008, 210–11; see Derrida 2001b, 27–28)

MATERNAL HIEROGLYPH

If paternity is a hieroglyph that requires interpretation, as Freud says following Lichtenberg, so too is maternity. The notion of a maternal hieroglyph as representative of chance, or *différance* itself, resonates with Julia Kristeva's rereading of Freud's interpretation of phobia, particularly animal phobia in children. In *Powers of Horror* (1980), Kristeva challenges Freud's hypothesis that the animal that terrifies (male) children represents their fathers. Reading the case of Little Hans, Kristeva argues that behind the paternal hieroglyph is a more opaque and indecipherable maternal hieroglyph. She claims that rather than representing paternal authority and the castration threat, the phobic "object" stands in for what cannot be adequately represented, especially by the child who is just learning language.

Little Hans's horse is a stand-in for complex psychic operations linked to separation from the maternal body and to learning to use words. Freud is certain that the animal phobias displace fears of the father and allow the child to continue loving him. For Kristeva, the fear is amorphous and cannot be so neatly anchored to the paternal function. Rather, the inability of words to adequately compensate for the loss of the maternal body produces a stand-in (the horse, wolf, or rat) for so many things that the child cannot represent, from its needs and desires to sensations of its body and the world around it. In her view, we are all phobic, trying to find the right words to reunite us with our lost love and a time before time and before the name or word.

Kristeva says of Little Hans, "the phobia of horses becomes a hieroglyph that condenses all fears, from unnamable to namable. From archaic fears to those that accompany language learning, at the same time as familiarization with the body, the street, animals, people. The statement 'to be afraid of horses,' is a hieroglyph having the logic of metaphor and hallucination. By means of the signifier of the phobic object, the 'horse,' it calls attention to the drive economy in want of an object—that conglomerate of fear, deprivation, and nameless frustration, which properly speaking, belongs to the unnamable" (1980, 33). Little Hans's horse becomes a living symbol of what is most commanding to Hans but also what he cannot name. Ultimately, for Kristeva this unnamable loss is associated with the maternal body, a maternal hieroglyph that stands in for the child's relation to the human condition as speaking animal (for a more detailed analysis of Kristeva on phobia, see Oliver 2009).

Kristeva also "revises" Freud's account in *Totem and Taboo* of the origin of representation from totemism and patricide. There, Freud gives another account of the move from prehistory where we existed as animals living merely by our senses in the primal horde to civilized society, which is enacted through the substitution of a representation of the father for the real father. Here again, he links representation to paternity and the substitutability of the father. I won't rehearse Kristeva's complex analysis. Suffice it to say that she finds matricide behind this patricide and again places her emphasis on the maternal body as what is behind representation, as a cipher for drives and affects as they make their way, always inadequately, into representation, through what she calls the semiotic. For my purposes, it is noteworthy that Kristeva suggests something like a maternal hieroglyph as an alternative to Freud's paternal hieroglyph. The maternal body as cipher stands in for—but never quite represents—relations to both parents, self and other, and inside and outside. It appears as a fluid threshold that haunts the psyche through the repeated return of the repressed. In her own way, Kristeva, like Derrida, challenges Freud's claim that representation begins with the paternal function. For Kristeva, it is much more complicated insofar as behind every terrifying father is an abject mother, who/that both threatens and enables representation and culture.

Deconstructive Genealogy

Discussing both the notion of paternal hieroglyph and Freud's story of the fraternal horde in *Totem and Taboo*, Derrida takes a different tack in deconstructing the paternal genealogy that is so certain for Freud. Again challenging Freud's attribution of sense-certainty to the mother (associated with physis) and representation to the father (associated with techne), Derrida argues that doubt is already present in the supposed plentitude of sense certainty postulated as our prehistorical origin, whether we are talking about Mother Nature or the "real" human-animal mother who gives birth. This uncertainty at the heart of maternal origins is made apparent by the possibility of surrogacy, where the maternal body as the body that bears the child may not be biologically related to the child; she could be a stranger, or the child's aunt, or grandmother, or sister, or a virgin. In addition, current technologies make it possible that the "biological mother" is unknown or anonymous, as in the case of anonymous egg donation, a complete stranger who contributes only a bit of genetic material. She could even be dead at the time of the child's birth. Although there are medical records, as Derrida reminds us, "there is no absolute archive, and the trace is not proof" (2004, 44).

In this time of ARTs, how do we know with certainty who is the mother or the father? Indeed, cloning makes it possible for the biological mother also to be the biological father, although until fetuses can be gestated outside of a woman's womb, it is unclear whether or not we can say that the biological father can also be the mother. Given these new technologies, what can we mean by *mother* or *father* anymore? The question, then, is not just who is the mother (or father). But rather, the question is what we can mean by *mother* or *father* in an age when conception can be outsourced, and multiple people can be involved in reproduction. This is the spirit of Derrida's deconstructive genealogy, which challenges not only the certainty of maternity but also of the very categories of kinship and genealogy so familiar to us:

> The deconstructive genealogy made possible and necessary through the "multi-mother," must retroactively spread through the concept of genealogy itself: which is a discursive or syntactical tool, interests, or phantasms and the history of institutions hidden behind them are stirred up, a deconstructive genealogy of this kind has to separate even those comfortable references which tie the representation, or rather the word of this genealogy to origin, to birth, the place of origin or birth, or the time. . . . The deconstructive genealogy of parenthood must also come into the discussion, which begins with the deconstruction of parenthood and straight through to the concept of conception. (1993b)

In light of deconstructive genealogy, how do we answer the question "who is the mother"? Is she the egg donor or the woman who carries the child and gives birth, what we call the "surrogate mother"? As we have seen, these new technologies lead to new forms of secrecy and testimony. Derrida argues, however, that they are not completely new, in that maternity, like paternity, has always been a matter of techne and testimony. They have never been "natural" and therefore "certain"—because this notion of nature, and Mother Nature (or natural mother) more specifically, is a fantasy, a fable, created as a result of a chain of substitute or surrogate mothers already operating in Her place. Her supposed eyewitness testimony also has been the testimony to something that cannot be seen. This something that cannot be seen is not only conception itself, but also and moreover the concept of motherhood. Our answer to the question "who is the mother?" is not an empirical fact that can be the matter of eyewitness testimony. Rather, it is a matter of a "legal fiction," or testimony of a different sort, testimony based on substitutability, replaceability, which is to say, surrogacy.

Deconstruction Has Always Been about Surrogacy

Derrida's analysis challenges us to consider the question "who is the mother?" not only in the literal or biological sense (egg donor, birth mother,

mother who raises the child), but also in the more radical sense of challenging our fixed concepts of mother, father, maternity, paternity, and family. Indeed, Derrida says, "deconstruction has always been 'of the family,' 'deconstruction of the family'" (2004, 37). Throughout his work, Derrida has revealed that conceptual tensions, fables, and legal fictions have always been at work in our traditional concepts of family. What we take to be mother, father, maternal, paternal, and family are shifty fictions rather than fixed origins. Although they may be the most familiar aspects of our experience, they are never obvious or transparent. They are never absolute or true in the ways that we imagine them to be. They always revolve around secrets, family secrets, which remain hidden, even hidden from their bearers in the deepest folds of the unconscious.

Most powerfully, our analysis of surrogacy reminds us that none of us are present at our own birth—or perhaps we should now say at our own conception—and therefore our parentage is always a fabulous fable. It is as if we are taught to repeat "mommy" and "daddy" over and over again in order to create maternity and paternity, those legal categories designated on our birth certificates where the "official" story is told. But as Derrida reminds us too, where there is official testimony there is also doubt, which is why official testimony is required at all. In one of the most fascinating parts of his interview with Roudinesco in *For What Tomorrow*, Derrida imagines that perhaps his parents are not who he thinks they are; and he asks what difference this would make: "I do believe that I know who my father and my mother were. And I can never know, with what is called certain knowledge, what happened between my presumed father and mother 'around' my birth. . . . [A]cts of deception (and other similar things—distraction and errors, multiple paths, complete misunderstandings, etc.) can suspend and hold at bay what you are calling the truth, what we desperately hope to maintain as the truth" (2004, 44–45). Imagining children switched at birth, he continues, "But if someone substitutes another child for theirs without their knowing it, if the secret is well kept, kept even from the unconscious, the parental bond will be established in the very same way. No one is any the wiser" (2004, 43). The point is not that accidents can happen and secrets are possible, but rather that there is an element of the accidental and the secret in all relations and all forms of reproduction, technologically enhanced or otherwise. Indeed, there is no otherwise to the technologically enhanced in any absolute way that opposes technology to nature or culture to biology. For all forms of reproduction, sexual or technological, involve techniques, supplements, and substitutions, perhaps most especially sex and family. And certainly, with the advent of anonymous sperm donors and egg donors, and other new reproductive technologies, including cloning, the accidents and secrets surrounding reproduction only multiply.

"Accidental" Pregnancy (Is There Any Other Kind?)

Derrida's deconstructive genealogy depends upon the deconstruction of physis and techne, which he repeatedly rehearses throughout his work. At this point, I would like to take my chances and reintroduce tyche into the mix, an element that is missing from Derrida's discussion of surrogacy. Indeed, in his essay "Who Is the Mother?" he traces certainty back to a fabulous maternal origin that is always already haunted by surrogates in the figures of "the foster mother, the wet nurse, ersatz mothers, the wide category of surrogate mothers." And in *For What Tomorrow*, he reminds us again of this series of mothers, and of Rousseau's substitute mothers in particular (2004, 41–42). Even before the appearance of the "real" surrogate mother, he says, "everything that we knew about the symbol of maternity would have been enough to undertake such work." But in what way is this work changed by the technological possibilities of new reproductive technologies? In what ways is it changed by the fact that there can now literally and biologically be "3+n" parents (cf. 2004, 37)? Derrida suggests that the paradox of testimony as "replication of the irreplicable" is the "paradox of our age." And he calls on the surrogate mother to witness to "the ancient intrusion of this technical prosthesis into physis." Yet he calls on her as always already a substitute mother, and therefore an interruption of the certitude accorded to the supposed eyewitness to birth. She is not the "real" mother, yet she gives birth. Is she even the *birth mother*? Not within current parlance, insofar as that term is reserved for the biological mother who gives her child up for adoption. So, what is she? And, more to the point in terms of Derrida's analysis, what does she witness?

In addition to the ancient technical prosthesis or replica at the heart of nature, doesn't she also witness to the accident of birth and the role of chance in both techne and physis? Derrida's account seems somehow too bloodless. Not in the sense of the fable or fantasy of blood relations that he says come "to be grafted—and to be nurtured like a parasite—on a fantasy of genetics: 'my flesh and blood!'; 'I love my child because he is my flesh and my blood, because he comes (a little) from me myself (a little, a little more) as another.' Well, I'm not so sure" (2004, 44). Rather, because the blood of birth is missing from his account. There are "rented wombs," "surrogate mothers," "gestational carriers," and "3+n parents," but where is the woman's experience of birth, whatever she may be to the child? Even if in a sense she is absent from the experience of birth (in so many ways, including drugs and the trauma that supposedly makes women "forget" or gives them "amnesia" afterwards), where is she in Derrida's testimony to the substitutability of the mother? While the mother may be substitutable, for the time being, birth is not—at least not in the sense that a woman still is required to give birth to that child of 3+n parents, and even to the clone.

Derrida asks us to consider a nongenealogical genealogy, a structure of parenthood as testimony that is not intergenerational insofar as "death or nonexistence is already in the heart of the living present." Yet this reinvention of *flesh and blood* through the surrogate as the container for mother-as-symbol discounts the "activity"—or perhaps I should say the *passivity*—of birth. However we answer the question "who is the mother?" and even if we defer it, we still run up against the fact that to this day all of us are born out of the body of a woman, which cannot be separated from whatever that may mean for us. To postulate either that the mother is an eyewitness who gives firsthand testimony from her natural privilege as present at birth, or to postulate that the mother is not an eyewitness but is already implicated in the structure of testimony as re-presentation, as compensation for lack or doubt (as Derrida does), cannot reach into the heart of birth as something that a woman does not control but rather undergoes. It is something that happens to her, and as such she is not present to it in the way that Derrida denies she is—or could we say, the way that he affirms it through his denial of it.

Moreover, what are we to make of the fact that even with birth control, most women who become pregnant without ARTs "do so" by "accident"? Indeed, what does it mean that we call unplanned pregnancy *accidental*? And in what sense can any pregnancy be *planned*? Even with ARTs, no one can say with certainty whether or not conception will take place, whether or not the embryo will "take" in the womb (which is why it is common to plant several embryos at once), or whether or not a baby will be born as a result. "Between the cup and the lip, many a slip," as they say. Indeed, it is standard practice to use "selective reduction" or abortion to reduce the number of viable embryos to one or two in cases where multiple embryos "take." Given that abortion is still a hot-button issue, this practice is usually kept quiet. And women rarely discuss it.

While Derrida uses the surrogate to deconstruct genealogies of certainty, and while the central notions of his deconstructive project revolve around chance, including *différance* and dissemination, he forgets about the role of chance and accident, tyche, in his discussions of surrogacy, ARTs, and cloning. The "accidental" nature of pregnancy already suggests that another even more unwieldy and chaotic element haunts the opposition between nature and culture or physis and techne—namely, chance. This is precisely what some contemporary discussions of ARTs, especially of genetic engineering and cloning, displace: the role of tyche (chance) in *both* physis (nature) and techne (technology). One of the ways that they do so is by erasing the role of the surrogate mother in these technologies. Here is where Derrida's deconstructive genealogy not only reminds us of the role of surrogacy in technologies of reproduction, but also reminds us that the question of technology is a question of reproduction that cannot skirt the surrogate.

Deconstructing Chance *versus* Control

Although current discussions of genetic engineering and cloning often turn on the triad *nature, technology, chance*, some strands displace chance onto nature and disavow its place in technology. Some contemporary bioethicists argue for replacing nature's haphazard evolutionary design with our own design—what Harris calls *enhancing evolution*—by taking matters into our own hands, eliminating chance in favor of control, and using nature to our own advantage as individuals and as a species. For example, Harris says, "I propose both the wisdom and the necessity of intervening in what has been called the natural lottery of life, to improve things by taking control of evolution and our future development to the point, and indeed beyond the point, where we humans will have changed, perhaps into a new and certainly into a better species altogether" (2007, 4–5). On this view, both human individuals and the species as a whole are better off if taken into hand through technology. Indeed, Harris goes so far as arguing that we have an ethical obligation to master our own biological and genetic destiny whenever possible. Clearly Harris prefers control to chaos; and he believes that technology helps us achieve this desired mastery over own our fate. Harris argues that technology gives us a way to control nature, particularly our own nature and thereby our own destiny.

What is telling in Harris's attitude toward technology is the relationship between order and chance as it operates in the relationship between nature and technology. Arguably, Harris accepts that biology is destiny, on the one hand, but insists on our ability to overcome that destiny, which is now figured as fate in the sense of chance rather than fate in the sense of biological determinism. Harris, it would seem, brings chance (tyche) back into the ancient triangle *physis, techne, tyche*. Whereas for the ancients both physis and techne are ordered and not a matter of chance, for Harris nature (physis) is a dicey gamble that requires technological intervention. Because I engaged Harris's arguments at length in the previous chapter, for now I use them as a foil in order to reveal a certain sleight of hand in their logic through my engagement with Derrida's deconstructive genealogy, specifically as it both reveals and conceals the role of tyche in both physis and techne.

Although a history—let alone a genealogy—of the relations between nature/physis, technology/techne, and chance/tyche is beyond the scope of this chapter, it seems widely accepted that in ancient discussions both nature and technology are seen as ordered by techne or craftsmanship, and both are opposed to tyche or chance. Plato and Aristotle, in radically different ways, believed that the order of nature (which Plato considered divine and Aristotle a matter of purposeful causes) was separate from the order imposed on nature by man. The difference in Aristotle's terms is between internal and external causes. For both Plato and Aristotle, man's relation to technology enables him to engage in purposeful creation and manufacture in terms of material, or matter, and ideas, or mind. For example, against the pre-Socratics, Plato insists that there is design or techne in nature (see *Sophist*, 265c), and Aristotle develops a complicated theory of nature or physis through which he articulates his theory of causes, while insisting that nature is ordered and teleological whether or not it is intelligent (cf. *Physics* 2, 199a). It is noteworthy that Seneca calls the active ordering principle in nature/physis *logos*, which he identifies with *logoi spermatikoi* (seminal reasons) on the level of the individual being (*De Beneficiis* 4, 7). For the Stoics, nature is associated with logos as *logoi spermatikoi* because it contains within itself the seeds of purposeful growth and diversity, which they saw as analogous to animal sperm (Von Arnim 2004, *Stoicorum Veterum Fragmenta*, 1:87 and 2:1027; Diogenes Laërtius 1925, *Lives of the Eminent Philosophers*, 7:135). For my purposes here, suffice it to say that for Plato and Aristotle both nature and technology are ordered and purposeful, and both are opposed to accident or chance/tyche, which is seen as inferior to either.

The valuation of control over chance, order over chaos, intentional over accidental, is precisely what is at stake in recent debates over genetic engineering and other new reproductive technologies (cf. Oliver 2010). What is fascinating in current discussions is how the dichotomy between technology and nature becomes one between chance and control, or chance and choice, where nature stands on the side of chance and technology on the side of control or choice. In other words, in contemporary debates, nature is no longer a matter of design or order but rather of accidents, randomness, and chance, or the "natural lottery of life." It seems that within bioethics, without a belief in a divine craftsman or first causes, physis is seen as ruled by tyche rather than by techne. Only man-made technology is truly a matter of craftsmanship because it begins and ends with purposeful human intervention, while nature, freed from a divine craftsman or telos, is a matter of chance and the randomness of natural evolution.

Even in the context of debates over genetic engineering in which presumptions of biological determinism undergird the discussion (for example, that DNA determines everything about us; that the mind is reducible to the brain; that biology is destiny), nature is associated with luck while technology is associated with purposeful ends. These discussions no longer revolve around whether both nature and technology are ordered, or how they might be ordered differently, but rather whether or not we should tamper with the uncertainties of the "lottery of life" and intervene with some measure of human control. More accurately, within these debates, it is usually a question of how much we should control, and not whether or not to control (in genetic engineering debates, even opponents of "positive eugenics" usually support some form of "negative eugenics"). In a sense, we could say that the *logoi spermatikoi* or seminal reasons are now literally within sperm itself and within other issues that contribute to reproduction, as long as they are put together by the master plan of a genetic engineer who carefully controls their dissemination.

Artificial Dissemination

Of course, Derrida has his own dissemination, which can offer a counterpoint to the dissemination of Harris's genetic engineer. Playing on the "fortuitous resemblance" between *seme* and *semen* (meaning and sperm), Derrida exploits this semantic "accident" to produce the "semantic mirage" not of insemination but rather of *dissemination*, dispersing surplus meanings, wasting the seed, extolling what he calls, in *Of Grammatology*, that "dangerous supplement" (1981, 45–46; cf. 1976). His concept of dissemination is intended to "interrupt" the illusion of plenitude and completeness that returns the son to the father and produces the fantasy of the proper legitimate heir. Returning to his analysis of Freud's old lady (who is a representative for Freud's mother, even his dead mother, or at least his fear of a dead mother), we find Derrida's engagement with the Freudian symptom as an accident that founds the certainty of psychoanalysis as a science. As Derrida points out, given Freud's account of the scientific certainty of the psychoanalytic enterprise, it is significant that the Greek *symptoma* also means "accident." Indeed, Derrida finds at the heart of the Freudian symptom an accident that links necessity, chance, and luck: "the marriage, as one would say in Greek, of Ananké, Tukhé, and Automatia" (2007, 350). A strange marriage this is, a *ménage à trois* of oppositional forces pulling in different directions, a precarious union or love triangle that makes nature predictable and determined, yet unpredictable, even random. Which is it then? Is nature ordered and necessary, or is it mere chance, even luck? Derrida maintains that the Greek *symptoma* operates in the "same semantic register" as "*the lottery*, of what is said to be attributed, distributed, dispensed, and sent (*geschickt*) by the gods or destiny . . . the chance of heredity, the play of chromosomes, as if this gift and these gifts obeyed, for better or worse, the order of a throw coming down from above. Destiny, destination: dispatches whose descending projection or trajectory can be disturbed, which in this case means interrupted or deviated" (2007, 350; my emphasis).

It is this lottery or accident of birth that bioethicists like Harris claim can be interrupted by human handiwork, which transforms chance into necessity through technology. On this view, human intervention into reproduction can lead to the end of symptoms, both in the sense of accidents of nature and in the sense of illness, since those who hold it believe that genetic engineering may eventually eliminate diseases and disabilities. Like the myriad philosophers whose disavowed and dead mothers Derrida reveals, and upon whose erased bodies they stake their claims to give birth to themselves, Harris and company completely ignore the fact that even clones have to be born out of the bodies of women, in which they gestate from embryos to viable fetuses and eventually babies (cf. Oliver 2012; O'Byrne 2010). Science fiction fantasies of adult clones being manufactured aside, surrogate mothers are still necessary even for the most advanced reproductive technologies (cf. Oliver 2012).

Why is this surrogate mother erased entirely from mainstream bioethics discussions of genetic engineering and other new reproductive technologies? Is it because she reintroduces chance into the world seemingly controlled by the scientist, doctor, or genetic engineer? Is it because she marks the place of the most fundamental disturbance to our way of thinking about ourselves as human beings conjured by new reproductive technologies? Is it because she interrupts technology as the return of repressed Mother Nature, that shadowy figure that has haunted the legitimate heirs to philosophy's mantle for centuries? Certainly her presence disturbs the fantasy of mastery so explicit in Harris's manifesto proclaiming the virtues of genetic engineering in terms of mastery over our destiny by controlling and thereby enhancing our own evolution. Perhaps more than any other figure, the surrogate mother reminds us that we are not, never have been, and never can be the masters of our own re-production. To think we can be is to disseminate a fable of human genealogy that once again discounts the role of the mother. It propagates the fantasy of man's triumph over the forces of Mother Nature through which he gives birth to himself without the body of woman/mother. This is the fable of technology—a fable that Derrida's deconstructive genealogy both reveals and conceals—namely, that through techne man overcomes both physis and tyche by erasing the flesh and blood of the maternal body altogether.

Parent or Patent?

Returning to the question with which we began—Does one invent the child?—we can extend Derrida's analysis of invention to ARTs and "designer babies." The dream that scientists and geneticists will someday control human reproduction, or perhaps the reproduction of everything on the planet, continues the dream of what Derrida calls phallologocentricism— namely, the dream that we can do away with both the mother and chance. This is a dream of absolute control and mastery that removes the mess of nature (including the maternal body) from the equation and substitutes the enhanced evolution of genetic science. Some see this as a dream, while others see it as a nightmare. In either case, the fantasy is one of control over what cannot be controlled, the chance and accidents that are the stuff of life. Throughout his work Derrida continually reminds us, "an accident can always happen" (e.g. 2002, 331). Moreover, all attempts to fix the opposition between the accidental and the necessary can be deconstructed.

Yet some philosophers such as Harris imagine making parents into patents, a possibility suggested too by the popular idiom *designer babies*. Derrida's discussion of surrogacy and cloning are instructive in this regard. But so too is his overall deconstructive project—and not just the deconstructive genealogy that he brings to the discussion of family—particularly in his discussion of nature versus culture, to which I return throughout this book. Derrida's analysis of invention is instructive in diagnosing what is happening in scientific, philosophical, and public policy debates over genetic engineering and ARTs, as practitioners on both sides try to calculate results and eliminate chance, not only to regulate but also to market and sell. ARTs are big business, and when it comes to business, usually gambles are taken only in order to make more profit. These practices attempt to overcome or abolish what Derrida calls the "aleatory event" in favor of predictable profit margins. Or, like John Harris, philosophers and scientists imagine futures where we have eliminated from human reproduction the natural lottery of life by replacing natural selection with deliberate selection.

The notion that we control or master chance (tyche) in either the realm of nature (physis) or of technology (techne) seems like hubris at best and outlandish, the stuff of science fiction, at worst. Yet Derrida's analysis does not turn on the empirical limitations that are disavowed in these debates— including the central one that I have highlighted, the disavowal of the fact that women are still required to gestate babies. Rather, his analysis turns on the conceptual tensions when we believe that we can invent the other, that we can invent the child. For, if invention is regulated and patented, then in what sense is it an invention of the other, rather than an invention of the same?[11] Specifically in terms of inventing the child, what would it mean to turn a parent into a patent?

We could say that this has been the aim of patriarchy all along: to make children into property. Of course, children were once legally considered the *property* of their fathers. And inheritance, as Derrida repeatedly reminds us, is about paternal *propriety* in a bond between fathers and sons through which the son inherits the *proper* name by virtue of the father's election or testimony. The father claims his rightful heir, while the son claims to be the rightful heir. And, in many cases, the courts must adjudicate competing claims. In a sense, Derrida attempts to expose patriarchy's matricidal fantasies that give the father privileged claims on the mother and *his* children as property, while at the same time preventing her, the mother, from becoming a substitute sovereign whose authority is just as absolute and tyrannical as hers (cf. Naas 2008).

Derrida's invocation of invention goes beyond what we might call these contaminated forms and toward an invention of the other as a pure invention (in the homeopathic sense, which I discuss in chapter 7), an invention of the other beyond calculation, predictions, control, or mastery. This is the chance we take. This is the chance that all parents take. Because whether or not the child is the result of ARTs or "good old-fashioned sex," its coming brings forth a future that is unpredictable. Indeed, the word *parent* is from the Latin *parere*, which means bringing forth. Bringing forth is not the same as bringing into being. It is not the same as creating *ex nihilo*. The etymology of the word *patent* is also instructive. For it not only means "conferring a title to sell," as well as "easily recognizable or obvious," but also "open and unobstructed." Indeed, *patent* is from the Latin *patere*, which means lying open.

What would it mean, then, to think of invention not in terms of the conferring of titles or proper names in an economy of property, not in terms of seeing oneself in one's offspring, obviously recognizable as one's own, but rather lying open to the otherness of the other, the otherness of the child to come? Can we imagine welcoming the future as a lying open to the "arrivingness" of the arrival, beyond our own control and mastery?

This is the deconstructive gesture that Michael Naas describes, "so as to think not exactly the mother but, perhaps, maternity—another name, here, for the event—anew, maternity without sovereignty and thus without phantasm, if there is such a thing" (2008, 211). Can we think parents as bringing forth and lying open to "the one who or which comes into one's home, and comes to oneself, inevitably, without invitation" (Derrida 2004, 59)? Whether the result of ART or not, can the birth of another be embraced with the Derridean gesture of welcoming the uninvited, the unannounced, and a gesture of pure hospitality that embraces what is always necessarily an aleatory event?

PART TWO

Medusa Machines

THREE

Girl Powered: Poetic Majesty against Sovereign Majesty

Recently we've seen a growing fascination with girls and wolves, whether it is the virgin high-schooler Bella Swan from *Twilight*, whose best friend turns out to be a werewolf, or sixteen-year-old virgin Katniss Everdeen from *The Hunger Games*, who hunts and kills wild dogs and other wild animals to feed her family and to have meat to trade for supplies, and is eventually chased by and forced to kill mutant wolves during the Hunger Games.[1] The title character of *Hanna* is another hunting virgin, trained by her father to fend for herself.[2] Indeed, all of these girls are tough as nails, fighting for their lives and killing when necessary. These are not your fairytale Little Red Riding Hoods, taken in by the Big Bad Wolf. Instead, they are mature beyond their years (Katniss); or, if a little naïve (Hanna), they are still killing machines who can take out the scariest wolf with one arrow (or maybe two). They are girls in danger, on the run, threatened; girls who rely on their wits to keep one step ahead of the baddies who want to kill them. They are both hunting and hunted. And in the cases of Katniss and Hanna, they have to learn to apply their hunting skills to killing people. Yet they are caught in between, not quite killers, but not innocent either; not quite good, but not bad either; not quite women, but no longer little girls. They appear to be natural girls, *sans* make-up, running through the woods; but they rely on techniques and technologies that they inherit from their fathers. Moreover, they are fantasies created for consumption by audiences hungry for strong female characters that aren't afraid to step out of their fathers' shadows, even if that means stepping into the shadow of the wolf. Not quite Athenas born from their fathers' heads, they metaphorically carry Athena's shield, evoking the threat of Medusa turning men to stone (or in Bella's case—after she eventually becomes a vampire—turning them to crystal and then to dust).

There are also virgin girls being pursued by wolves, both enraging their virility and challenging it, in Jacques Derrida's *The Beast and the Sovereign*, volume 1 (2009). In this chapter I explore the role played by the figure of the virgin girl at the center of that text.[3] She may offer a figure between the beast and the sovereign, between the two machines (or marionettes) of nature and culture. Moreover, she not only props up the fabled distinction between man and animal, but also is that upon which man erects himself as sovereign lord and master. Taking Derrida's suggestions further, I argue that the virgin girl both does and undoes sovereign power as phallic power. She is the figure behind the erection of sovereignty. Her unveiling as such— what we could call the deflowering of the fable of deflowering virginity— reveals the phallus itself to be a puppet, a marionette, not exactly under her control but certainly not under man's control either. Indeed, her appearance is both necessary and threatening insofar as she both erects sovereign phallic power and threatens to reveal its impotence. In this way, the girl operates between feminine and masculine, between nature and culture, between the beast and the sovereign, particularly as her virginity and its deflowering are essential to the cut between the two sides of these traditional binaries. Furthermore, in Derrida's engagement with Celan, the appearance of the girl is vital to his discussion of art and representation.[4] And her appearance is telling in relation to the movements and rhythms of Derrida's deconstructive approach to philosophy and literature in *The Beast and the Sovereign* and in his work more generally. Finally, following Elizabeth Rottenberg's Little Red Riding Hood as she moves through Derrida's text,

I conclude where I began, with role reversals between the girl and the wolf, possibly to the point of deconstructing the girl-wolf opposition.

The Set-Up (the Con)

After playing with various wolf idioms and foreshadowing a few of the wolves to come, ranging from those of Hobbes to those of La Fontaine, Derrida insists, "When I say wolf, you mustn't forget the she-wolf . . . often a symbol of sexuality or even of sexual debauchery or fecundity" (2009, 9). Yet in spite of this reminder, he does not return to the she-wolves of intellectual history, preferring to focus on the ways in which political man is figured like a wolf, although sexual difference is often explicit and always implicit in his formulation of the beast (feminine) and the sovereign (masculine). Derrida begins the first lecture of *The Beast and the Sovereign* with the words "Feminine . . . masculine [La . . . le]" (2009, 1). This is a phrase that he repeats at the opening of many of these lectures, a phrase that circulates throughout the seminar. Starting here, he remarks that the feminine beast and the masculine sovereign form a couple, marking not only sexual difference but also an "alliance or hostility, war or peace, marriage or divorce," and already "going at each other," "making a scene" (2). His very next move is to invoke the figure of the wolf, not only to suggest that he will "creep up" on the topic of the beast and the sovereign and their alliance/ hostility rather than address it head-on, but also to ask his audience to keep in mind figures of the wolf running throughout political philosophy and the Western imaginary.

The sovereign is usually the wolf, or the biggest *baddest* wolf—the alpha male—that keeps all of the other wolves at bay (as we know from Freud and Levi-Strauss, usually fighting over the women). Interestingly, while the animal is never far from the feminine (given the associations between women and animals in the history of Western thought), the beast, the beastly, the *bêtise* that come to occupy the seminar revolve around man's inhumanity to man, man's cruelty that is more beastly than that of any beast. This notion of man's beastliness and his stupidity (*bêtise*) repeatedly marks his uniqueness within the animal kingdom and comes to define the man-animal divide. Analyzing texts from Aristotle, Hobbes, Bodin, Lacan, Deleuze, and Agamben, along with poems by Celan and Lawrence, among others, Derrida demonstrates how the opposition between the human and the animal comes back to something beastly, not just the beastliness and stupidity of that opposition in the first place, but also the various ways in which it shows itself throughout these varied texts as a matter of the beastliness or stupidity (*bêtise*) of man.

Bêtise becomes not just one distinction among others, but a type of transcendental signifier of the linguistic difference supposedly reserved for mankind (cf. 2009, 151; 167). Derrida spends much time explaining how the French word *bétise* has no simple translation that captures all of its meanings. In French it has no univocal meaning; rather its meaning must be determined by its context (162). Yet Derrida suggests that the multiple meanings of this word do not make its meaning undecidable in the same way as the meanings of other complicated words. It is not just that its meaning cannot be determined apart from its context, but also and moreover that the stakes when it comes to the man-animal divide are all about determinability versus indeterminability, dumb versus having the capacity for speech (cf. 173). At stake in the undecidability of the meaning of this word, *bêtise*, is the very ability to decide, which has been reserved for man and denied to animals.

Sovereignty, then, is what is at stake in who or what is *bêtise* or *bête*. Who has sovereignty and what does not. Who can decide and what cannot. Who and what. This is another phrase that Derrida repeats. To be *who* is already to have it; to be *what* is to have it not.

Enter the marionette, the machine, the absolute *what* against which all other whats (and whos) are measured.[5] Remember Descartes's conclusion that animals are machines: they are machines in that they are determined, their behavior decided by nature, while humans are free, able to decide for themselves; animals are governed by natural laws, while humans have invented culture and govern themselves. Derrida asks what is more automatic, more mechanistic, more beastly—nature or culture, unconscious behavior or conscious behavior?

> Fascination, fetishization, consciousness or unconscious projections: what is less *bête* or more *bête*, more or less cunning, consciousness or unconsciousness? Each says, both say to each other, one is more *bête* than the other. This undecidable alternative, both "strange and familiar," uncanny, *unheimlich*, would go just as well for life and death, the living and the dead, the organic and the inorganic, the living being and the machine, the living being and its

mechanization, the marionette, the mortal and the immortal: one is always more *bête* than the other. The truth of *bêtise* is no doubt this reciprocal upping of the ante, this denying hyperbole that always adds *bêtise*, a supplement of *bêtise*, to the self-proclamation of its opposite. (2009, 184)

Has the she-wolf, or at least a foxy woman, crept back into Derrida's articulation of this question of consciousness versus unconsciousness as one of the cunning and uncanniness of marionettes or machines? Derrida suggests as much. First, in his explanation that the meaning of the French words *bête* and *bêtise* are determined by their context, he introduces another difficult French word, *con*, which means "bloody idiot" but also is obscene slang for female genitalia (cf. 169). Second, his use of the German word *unheimlich* to designate the uncanny recalls Freud's use of the term in relation to female genitalia; even in the context of Derrida's explicit reference to Paul Celan's speech, "The Meridian," *unheimlich* is related to the site of girls and the figure of Medusa. And third, as he points out, the word *marionette* comes from *mariolette*, a miniature representation of the Virgin Mary (188).

Derrida gives a new twist to the relation between consciousness and unconsciousness by asking which is most beastly (most animal and/or most cruel). He answers that each says to the other that it is the most beastly. The split between conscious and unconscious—and thereby, response and reaction, free and determined—which is definitive for man is dependent upon what he calls *upping the ante* with the supplement of beastliness or *bêtise*. In other words, the supplement of *bêtise* is the ultimate insult in that it not only accuses one side of the divide or the other of being stupid or animal, but also and moreover both forecloses the possibility of the animal ever being included in the moral community or civil society on one side, and the possibility of free will or liberty in what we take to be that community on the other. Indeed, its foreclosure is simultaneously the condition of possibility of the moral community and civil society, and what makes the moral community and civil society impossible.

The way that Derrida articulates a certain paradox here between the possibility of free will and moral choices and their impossibility is a hallmark of his deconstructive method. In a related discussion in *The Animal that Therefore I Am* (2008), he makes a similar move when he suggests that either animals can be included on the culture side of the nature-culture divide, or humans cannot be properly included there. In other words, animals may not be as *bête* as we think they are, on the one hand, and we may be more *bête* than we claim, on the other. There, he argues that everything we take to be proper to the human, everything that we take to be distinctive of humanity, is not fully or properly our own; or at least we can never be certain that it is. For example, can we be certain that our actions are determined by neither biology nor culture? Can we be certain that our decisions are freely chosen and not influenced by factors outside of our control, such as language, tradition, cultural values, not to mention bodily impulses, drives, or DNA?

But what does it mean to ask whether the conscious mind or the unconscious body is more *bête* or more *con*? In *The Beast and the Sovereign*, Derrida's answer to this question appears between "two *arts of the marionette*, two marionettes, whose fables intersect" (2009, 188). In making this provocative claim, Derrida, as he does so often throughout his work, identifies a supplement at the heart of what we take to be original or natural, both to the animal beast and to the human sovereign. The operation of this supplement is "a question of art, of *tekhne* as art or of *tekhne* between art and technique, and between life and politics" (187). He claims that "a prosthetic supplement" "comes to replace, imitate, relay, and augment the living being" (187). Moreover, he argues that this supplement not only replaces the original, but also comes first and creates the original, or the illusion of an origin, of nature in itself. This act of reproduction cannot be easily distinguished from an act of production, and vice versa. But what is clear is that *techne* or art is at the center of what we take to be natural and original. To accuse either nature with its unconscious bodies or culture with its conscious minds of being *bête* is to expose the fiction or fable upon which their "natures" are produced. Another way of asking the question with which we began is: Which is the biggest con, the fable of nature or of culture?

This is where the marionette comes in. The marionette (what we could call the machine) is fabled not to control itself but rather to be controlled by the marionette master. But who is its master, and how can we be so sure that *he* controls the puppet and not the other way around? Or that whoever or whatever is pulling the strings can be known to man, let alone controlled by man? Just as the machine seems to need an operator, and art or technology assume an agent, so too does the marionette with its master. By engaging with various texts throughout the history of philosophy, particularly political philosophy, along with some literary texts across genres (including novels, poetry, fables, and a speech), Derrida teases out the operations of art and technology that cannot be controlled or mastered, most especially by what we take to be human agency, or what traditionally has been called *man*. The operations of art and technology, like the operations of these various texts, take us well beyond the control of their supposed authors. Indeed, they are always doing more than their authors know or intend, assuming of course that their authors know or intend anything that can be identified for certain, which is also put into question. Derrida is not arguing for fatalism or that everything is determined on both sides of the nature-culture binary. He is claiming that there is mechanization on both sides; both sides operate according to the *fabular*, even fabulous, logic of the supplement; and neither side escapes the uncanny effect of prosthesis. In this way, he also deconstructs the opposition between freedom and determinism, and thereby the very question of the possibility of making a sovereign decision becomes undecidable: "this undecidable alternative, both 'strange and familiar,' uncanny, *unheimlich*, would go just as well for life and death, the living and the dead, the organic and the inorganic, the living being and the machine, the living being and its mechanization, the marionette" (2009, 184).

The Uncanny Effect of Mothers and Girls

The figure of the marionette comes to represent the uncanniness of this undecidability between life and death, organic and inorganic, freely chosen or mechanistically determined. Although Derrida doesn't mention Freud's essay on the uncanny, it haunts his discussion of the marionette. For in that essay, the most chilling example of the uncanny effect is in Hoffmann's "The Sandman," which is the story of young Nathaniel falling in love with Olympia, whom he only ever sees from afar through the window. He becomes terrified when he realizes one day that the girl he has admired is really a doll, an automaton, a marionette. The uncanny effect is created when something that should be inanimate becomes animated or vice versa, like the Olympia marionette, a lifelike double for a real girl. She is so lifelike that Nathaniel falls in love with her. As I mentioned earlier, in this same essay Freud concludes that the ultimate representative of the uncanny is the mother's sex, particularly insofar as it also represents both life and death (according to Freud); it is the original home, and yet—or perhaps for that reason—also terrifying. The horror of the female genitals is a recurring theme for Freud, which is perhaps nowhere more apparent than in two of his essays that Derrida does cite in his discussion of the marionette, namely "Medusa's Head" and "The Taboo of Virginity" (cf. 2009, 223). In those two essays, Freud argues that the female sex is both fascinating and terrifying because it signals castration; that is, the male sees the female sex as castrated and fears that it may castrate him. As we return to Derrida's discussion of the uncanny marionette as a figure for art, keep in mind Freud's essays on the threat of castration posed by the female sex.

In *The Beast*, Derrida plays between two marionettes, one in Valéry's *Monsieur Teste* and the other in Celan's "The Meridian" (cf. Derrida 2011, 78–79). The opening words of the latter are: "Ladies and Gentlemen, Art, you will remember, has the qualities of the marionette and the iambic pentameter. Furthermore—and this characteristic is attested in mythology, in the story of Pygmalion and his creature—it is incapable of producing offspring" (quoted in Derrida 2009, 185).[6] Derrida comments on what "remains unheimlich" about art, what Celan describes as a circular movement both strange and familiar, both traveling and homecoming, a liberating encounter that requires "rabbit's ears" to listen "not without fear, for something beyond itself, beyond words" (Celan 2003, 54). Derrida hears the uncanny and inhuman in Celan's description of art, represented by figures of Medusa's head, the monkey, and the marionette and other automatons. Celan concludes, "Art (this includes Medusa's head, the mechanism, the automaton), art, the uncanny strangeness which is so hard to differentiate and perhaps is only *one* after all—art lives on." Art, "this road of the impossible," leads to a *meridian*, the highpoint of life, beyond humanity; it leads to an uncanny encounter with life's breath itself (Celan 2003, 52, 54–55). Beyond the human, toward the inhuman, the animal (monkey), the machine (marionette), Derrida provocatively invokes the impossible place or space "between two marionettes," between the beast (*la*-feminine) and the sovereign (*le*-masculine). We could also say between nature and culture, or between the ancient notions of *physis* and *techne*.

Here, once again, as he has done so many times throughout his work, Derrida locates *techne*, or artifice, at the heart of nature or origin. What we take to be original is really a copy, a supplement, after all. As he does in

Of Grammatology with the figure of the mother and mother-nature in Rousseau, Derrida shows how art and artifice create the fiction of origin, which depends upon them to function as such. Like Rousseau, Pygmalion creates his substitute woman. She is a fiction created through artifice. She is the product of his imagination, an object of art, and as such is not flesh and blood. She is a marionette and not a real girl. No real woman is good enough for him, so he creates one of his own, his property, his projection. She (like art—and perhaps clones) cannot reproduce and remains childless; and therefore so does Pygmalion, unless you count her as his child, his stone beloved, born from his own head, but not of woman born. Ultimately, the ideal woman is a fiction, a creation that engenders the original. Moreover, what Derrida's deconstructive apparatus suggests is that what we take to be the "real girl" is also a fable. Yet at the same time he seems to insist that flesh and blood, some really real girl, cannot be written. Perhaps the real girl is like the real cat that he does not, and cannot, name in *The Animal that Therefore I Am*, because to name her already is to kill her. To name her is already to re-present her and therefore to lose her. She is always in excess of any attempt to name her, to describe her, to reproduce her. She is beyond reproduction and yet what engenders it. Perhaps the real girl, like the real cat, is not liberated by poetry or art but rather escapes it, runs ahead of it, and is always out of its grasp.

Derrida's engagement with Celan's "The Meridian" revolves around a passage involving girls escaping art that belongs to a text by Georg Büchner, quoted by Celan in this speech accepting the Büchner Prize. Derrida quotes Celan at length; or more accurately, Derrida quotes Celan quoting Büchner's *Lenz* fragment (an homage to Reinhold Lenz), which I now quote here:

> "Yesterday, as I was walking along the edge of the valley, I saw two girls sitting on a rock; one was putting up her hair and the other was helping; and the golden hair was hanging down, and the face, pale and serious, and yet so young, and the black dress, and the other one so absorbed in helping her. The most beautiful, the most intimate of pictures of the Old German School can convey but the vaguest impression of such a scene. At times one might wish to be a Medusa's head so as to be able to transform such a group into stone, and call out to the people."
>
> Ladies and Gentlemen, please take note: "One would like to be a Medusa's head," in order to . . . comprehend that which is natural as that which is natural, by means of art! . . .

Here we have stepped beyond human nature, gone outward, and entered
an uncanny realm, yet one turned toward that which is human, the same realm
in which the monkey, the automata, and accordingly . . . alas, art, too seem to
be at home. (Quoted in Derrida 2009, 185–86; cf. Celan 2003, 42)

Here is a scene of two girls who appear deeply embedded in the discourses of several men (Derrida, Celan, Büchner, Lenz), who call upon the
girls to make a point about the relation between art and nature, between
techne and physis. The two girls, held in the gaze of a man who sees them
without being seen—what Derrida calls the *visor effect*—invoke Medusa,
another girl with hair hanging down (not lucky enough to have kept her
head so that she too could put up such unruly hair).[7] The Medusa's head
would allow the artist to freeze these young girls absorbed by their
intimate, innocent touching, and to bring others over to see nature in all
of its beauty. For his part, the artist, here the poet or author, can only
describe the scene using words, then indicate how even the greatest Old
German masters could not imitate such a scene, and describe his wish for a
Medusa's head, not to wield it like a brush but to become it in order to be
the agent of these girls' turning to stone. Only the power of Medusa's
head could freeze the girls in this moment of undisturbed concentration on
their task.

The Medusa Effect

In the essay "Medusa's Head," Freud interprets the horrifying aspect of the
Medusa's head as the terror of castration evoked by this representative of
female genitals—open-mouthed, surrounded by hair, frequently figured
as snakes, which displace the penis and thereby both trigger and mitigate
the horror of castration. Freud says, "The sight of the Medusa's head makes
the spectator stiff with terror, turns him to stone. Observe that we have
here once again the same origin from the castration complex and the same
transformation of affect! For becoming stiff means an erection. Thus in
the original situation it offers consolation to the spectator: he is still in
possession of a penis, and the stiffening reassures him of the fact" ([1922]).
Although Derrida uses the Medusa's head in the context of discussing the
uncanny effects of art, framed by an insistence on the sexual difference
implicit in the pair *beast* (la-feminine) and *sovereign* (le-masculine), neither

he nor Celan comment on Büchner's account of Lenz's desire for Medusa's head as the invocation of another girl, or even of a set of girls, as protection against the innocence of two girls engaged in their own desires without concern for the man watching them and the effects of their display of intimacy on him. Medusa is one of three girls, three sisters, the Gorgons, who are animal-woman hybrids with wings and snakes for hair. Medusa is also the protector of Athena, the virgin goddess, who wears the Medusa's head on her dress to repel sexual desire by displaying "the terrifying genitals of the Mother" (Freud [1922]). Medusa is another she-wolf insofar as she represents the uncanny effects of the mother's sex, sexual and fecund, attractive and terrifying, castrated and reassuring.

In Freud's analysis, the Medusa's head not only represents the castration of the female sex but also reassures the male that he is not castrated, and moreover that he is potent when he stiffens in her presence. The dual result—both threatening castration by representing castration/decapitation and mitigating against the castration threat by representing the multiplication of the penis/hair and stiffening the spectator—further extends Medusa's uncanny effect. Again, Freud quickly moves from the decapitated/castrated Medusa to the erect male organ as a repellant or apotropaic act; he says, "to display the penis (or any of its surrogates) is to say: 'I am not afraid of you. I defy you. I have a penis'" ([1922]). This virile display is an act intended to intimidate through phallic power. This is one of the structures of sovereign power that Derrida challenges, namely, sovereignty as the assertion of power through virile display. This form of sovereignty is not only evident in the history of political philosophy and in the history of politics, but also in contemporary struggles for political power and current political discourse.

Derrida argues that this type of sovereignty is always a *performance* of sovereignty, always the assertion of power legitimating itself by putting on the show of power. Political sovereignty as the "right of the stronger" and of the most virile is on display in La Fontaine's fable "The Heifer, the Goat, and the Ewe in Society with the Lion," which Derrida quotes to make his point. There, the lion claims the right to all four parts of a stag, giving reasons why he should have each part: the first he claims because of his capacity as Sire and the fact that he is called *Lion*, the second because he is the strongest, the third because he is the most valiant, and the fourth because, as he says, "if any one of you girls touches the fourth, I'll strangle her right now" (quoted in Derrida 2009, 213). Here again are three girls, three sisters, kowtowing to the lion because he is a Sire and therefore stronger. His sovereignty, his majesty as lion, is a performance through which he asserts that *might makes right*. He says he is the strongest and threatens to strangle the girls if they object. Derrida argues that this is not only a lesson in how sovereign power works, as *might makes right*, but also a lesson in how it works as fictional and performative. This type of sovereign power is itself a fable told by the "strongest" in order to assert his "right" to rule.

The story also provides another example of sovereignty propped up by the invocation of girls. In Derrida's-Celan's-Büchner's *Lenz*, the sight of girls provokes the violent fantasy of a decapitated Medusa with snakes for hair that turns the girls to stone. In the fable of the lion, the Sire threatens to strangle the girls if they challenge his rights, or, on Derrida's reading, his fable or story of rights. Yet the girls are necessary witnesses to the lion's performance. For a performance is nothing without an audience. And the girls are necessary to the lion's claim; they are the audience for his fable. Moreover, the three girls are necessary characters in La Fontaine's fable. And this repetition of the appearance of girls in Derrida's own fable about the relationship between the beast and the sovereign suggests that they play a central role there too. We could say that these girls, or the figure of the girl—like the animal or the machine—become what in *Of Grammatology* (1976) Derrida calls *nicknames* for the operation of *différance* always in excess of the categories it may produce. In this way, the girl is a figure for what is in excess of the binary opposition between the beast and the sovereign, the feminine and the masculine, or nature and culture (the two marionettes). We could say that she is a figure for what Derrida educes as "between two marionettes": "What if the [feminine] marionette were between the two, between the two marionettes—between the *who* and the *what*—both sensible and insensible, neither sensible nor insensible, sensible-insensible . . . sensible insensible, living dead, spectral, uncanny, *unheimlich*?" (2009, 187).

We even could go further to suggest that both mothers and girls are uncanny because they fall outside of sexual difference, or fall between two marionettes, insofar as neither is identical with the category *woman* or the category *feminine*. In a sense, they are the before and after of these categories, particularly as seen from the perspective of patriarchal culture. Both remind man that he cannot reproduce by himself. When he tries, he ends up like Pygmalion, in love with a piece of stone and childless. This is not to say that the mother or the girl is not circumscribed by cultural constructs or fantasies. To the contrary, they both are marionettes, so to speak, insofar as their strings are pulled by social conventions. Both the mother and the girl, even more than the woman or the feminine, are associated with biology over culture and are thereby caught between two marionettes, nature and culture. Returning to Derrida's text, we could say that the figure of the girl props up or erects the fabled distinction between the beast (la-feminine/nature) and the sovereign (le-masculine/culture), and at the same time she is that upon which he props himself up or erects himself as sovereign. Tracking the movements of Derrida's marionettes through his engagement with Valéry's *Monsieur Teste* will further substantiate this interpretation.

Could a Woman Hold This Discourse?

In his discussion of Valéry, Derrida comments on the character of M. Teste, who insists that he has killed the marionette within himself by distancing himself both from his bodily appetites and from cultural conventions; for both nature and culture are capable of turning him into a marionette, reacting to something out of his control rather than controlling his body and his actions via his reason and intellect. Through a subtle and detailed engagement with Valéry's text, Derrida concludes:

> There are only doubles of marionettes here, and it's difficult to know who controls them, who is the boss, the author, the creator or the sovereign, the manipulator and puppeteer. Just as it is difficult to know what a marionette is, if it is something of the order of the mechanical and inanimate thing (reacting without responding, to pick up our Cartesian-Lacanian distinction again), or if it is of the order of an animated, animal thing (a living being of pure reaction presumed to be without speech and responsible thought), or if it is already of the human order, and thereby able to emancipate itself, to respond autonomously, as it were, and to take hold, prosthetically, prosthstatically, of a sovereign power. (2009, 189)

In this analysis of M. Teste's desire to kill off the marionette within himself, Derrida asks whether we can imagine killing something that is already dead; what would it mean to kill off the marionette, especially the marionette within oneself, to kill off everything that is automatic in oneself, whether it be animal instinct or cultural ritual? What would it mean to kill off the animal-machine, the being speaking? *Who* could do it? *Who* or *what* would be left after such elimination? Derrida suggests that this animal-machine reproduces itself with a "pigheaded stubbornness" that cannot be overcome even when its adversary is the arrogant M. Teste. Derrida points out that M. Teste's name itself brings to mind the head of this pigheadedness, the *tête*, along with testicles and testimony—we are already back to the question of reproduction, and therefore of women. M. Teste claims only to have "touched on women" without actually being touched by them (2009, 197). We might wonder, in passing, how much Derrida has touched on women in his texts and how much he has been touched by them. For it is curious that although Derrida is aware of feminist concerns and attends to issues of sexual difference throughout his work, he rarely discusses texts by women. In other words, where do we locate sovereignty in his texts? Who is doing the touching and who is being touched?

In this animal-machine that stubbornly reproduces itself with an instinct too strong to overcome, the she-wolf has returned once again. For in Derrida's brief mention of her, she seems to represent preprogrammed instincts, on the one hand, and sexual agency, on the other. She is a figure for dangerous reproductive instincts out of control, and for dangerous sexual agency run rampant. She is both determined by natural instincts beyond her control, and the agent or sovereign of a dangerous sexuality that can be wielded by her against males. Like the praying mantis or black widow spider, in this way, the she-wolf is another representative of what is uncanny about the mother's sex, particularly as it signals female sexuality and/as fecundity, as out of men's control and therefore threatening to them.

Recall that early in *The Beast and the Sovereign*, Derrida warns us not to forget that the she-wolf is always in the background of the seminar: "When I say wolf, you mustn't forget the she-wolf. What counts here is no longer the sexual difference between the wolf as a real animal and the mask [*loup*] worn by the woman. Here we are not dealing with this double wolf, this 'twin' word, masculine in both cases, the natural wolf, the real wolf and its mask *le loup*, its simulacrum, but indeed with the she-wolf, often a symbol of sexuality or even of sexual debauchery or fecundity, of the she-wolf mother" (2009, 9). Derrida insists that the she-wolf is neither the real wolf nor its mask, but rather the she-wolf is a figure for dangerous female sexuality and fecundity. He suggests that she is beyond sexual difference as set up in the twin meanings of the French word *loup*, wolf and mask (worn by women). How might this symbol of female sexuality, even debauchery, and fecundity be beyond sexual difference? What is Derrida saying when he maintains that sexual difference does not count here? Is he perhaps suggesting that the wolf, the mask, and the she-wolf as trope or figure are all on the side of the masculine, or projections of masculine desire? Or is he merely suggesting that although sexual difference is relevant, it doesn't count when we are dealing with a figure for fecundity or motherhood? In other words, maternal and paternal are not the same as feminine and masculine; although they are related to sexual difference, they cannot be reduced to it. Or could Derrida be suggesting that the she-wolf is between the feminine and the masculine in the same way as is the marionette? Could the she-wolf ever be Little Red Riding Hood? Indeed, could the she-wolf devour Little Red's grandmother and assume her place? Could the fabulous wolf so familiar to us from children's fables (and political philosophy) be a she-wolf after all? Could Little Red Riding Hood and the Big Bad Wolf be one and the same?

These questions resonate with Derrida's provocative question, "Could a woman hold this discourse?" referring to that master's discourse of M. Teste (2009, 188). Again, we could ask the same question of Derrida's own discourse (especially when we get to the suggestion that the temporality of deconstruction operates according to the phallic rhythms of erection and detumescence). Derrida asks this question of M. Teste's discourse of killing off everything that is automatic in himself, most especially the ways in which his actions are determined by his body and social conventions. He puts himself above both nature and culture to declare his own sovereign self as master of everything beastly in himself. Could a woman declare her independence from her body and the traditions that link her to animality? Could she absolve herself from the image of her sexuality and fecundity as that of a she-wolf? Could a woman, who by those cultural constructs is associated with the contaminating influence of the body, say that she has only "touched on women," and that she has killed off the woman in herself? Could she assert her absolute independence from both the animal and from all others, including the laws and rituals of culture? Derrida asks,

"Could a woman hold this discourse? And say *'La bêtise n'est pas mon fort'* [Stupidity is not my strong suit] as her first words, as soon as she opens her mouth," as does M. Teste (188; translation modified)? What happens when she tries?

Sarah Palin, Mama Grizzly, She-Wolf par Excellence

Enter Sarah Palin. Imagine the effect of Sarah Palin saying, "Stupidity is not my strong suit." Think of Sarah Palin, who is "going rogue" and loving it. She adopted the Republican Party's image of her as a rogue elephant that does not accept her place in the herd. She is a "mama grizzly," a lipstick-wearing "pit bull," protecting family values (if not her own children). She holds this discourse through the fable of killing the Big Bad Wolf of big government, protecting Little Red Riding Hood (even if this little girl already has been knocked up by some other little wolf). She is the phallic mother, both threatening to castrate the political establishment and at the same time propping up phallic power, even patriarchal power, by performing her motherhood, femininity, and most especially sexy celebrity status. More appropriately, then, we might say that she is a fetishized replacement for the phallic mother, who like the figure of Priapus with his permanent erection, mentioned by Derrida, is both threatening and comic. The fertility god Priapus's permanent erection is ridiculous and funny, especially because, despite his huge erection, he is impotent. So too it is funny when a sexy woman puts on phallic political power and flaunts it on stage, wink, wink. When Palin straps on phallic power her performance demonstrates how political power as phallic power is about the performance of macho virility. How funny is a permanent erection when wielded by a ravenous, meat-loving, beast-killing beauty queen, queen-bee-cum-political-figure trying to prove she's nobody's puppet? Sarah Palin, who says there is room for all of Alaska's animals . . . right next to the mashed potatoes. With her image as a moose-killing, baby-popping, Harley-riding, tough-love kinda all-American gal, you betcha she is more macho than the macho men.

In the age of televisual media, Derrida argues that "all political leaders, heads of state, or heads of parties, all the supposedly decisive and deciding actors of the political field are consecrated as such by the election of their erection to the status of marionette in the puppet show . . . the most significant thing being the desire of said notables to be elected to this erection to the status of marionettes. Election to the erection" (2009, 216). Derrida gives as his example of this phenomenon the *Bébête Show*, a French puppet show modeled on *The Muppets* that had politicians appear in the form of animal puppets. Today, politicians regularly appear on comedy shows to spoof themselves, erecting themselves as marionettes in hopes of election to the erection as sovereign. Think of Sarah Palin's memorable appearance on *Saturday Night Live* during the 2008 presidential election, when she was shown be-bopping to Amy Poehler's singing about killing and skinning a moose. Sarah Palin between two marionettes, who performs both the beast and the sovereign: She is that jumble of contradictory stereotypes all rolled into one iconic figure, the Phallic Mother, only now sexier than ever, our new fetish. Sarah Palin the MILF, as the marionette who performs political election as political erection; or who at least plays with her erectablity, if not her electability. Sarah Palin the political animal, sexy ex-governor, foxy politician, or crazy-like-a-fox she-wolf par excellence.

Girl on a Stick, or, The Phallic Law of the Marionette

By asking, "The phallus, I mean the *phallos*, is it proper to man?" Derrida forces us to ask not just whether a woman can hold this discourse, but also whether a man can hold it (2009, 206). Can he keep it up? Can His Majesty the Sovereign maintain his erection? And what happens when he tries? Derrida answers, "This standing, erect, augmented grandeur, infinitely upped, this height superior to every other superiority is not merely a trope . . . but an essential feature of sovereign power, an essential attribute of sovereignty, its absolute erection, without weakness or without detumescence, its unique, stiff, rigid, solitary, absolute, singular erection" (215). The performance of erection is essential to election. And yet who can maintain this act, this fable of sovereign power? Who can permanently erect himself by making his platform and therefore his vantage point the highest, the grandest, the most? Derrida deconstructs these grand platforms by exposing them as simulacra, prostheses, wooden legs, or, we might say, wooden woodies. And again, who or what is behind this woody, this performance of the erection of sovereign power? Here, what gives rise to Derrida's extended discussion of erection is that group of girls of La Fontaine's fable, the heifer, the goat, and the ewe. And it is through the girl, this time the virgin, that Derrida connects the erection and the marionette.

Derrida reminds us that the figure of the marionette is herself a figurine of "the small and the young, the little girl, the touching innocent girl, even the virgin, the Virgin Mary (*mariole*, *mariolette*). With the grace, innocence, and spontaneity that usually go with that" (2009, 220). But no sooner does he recall us to this figure of innocence that comes to represent both the possibility and impossibility of the relation between art and nature, than he warns, "but as you have no doubt already sensed, things are not so simple. In truth, they are less simple than ever. As always when sexual differences are in play" (220). Immediately, however, (although only parenthetically), Derrida issues another warning about his warning, even commenting on his propensity for issuing warnings—or more accurately, he issues a warning about those who are suspicious of his warnings, those who do not take his warnings to heart: "I believe it's primarily because they want to hide from themselves, forget or deny something to do with sexual differences. There's always a clandestine debate raging about sexual differences" (220). Yet the figure of the girl as marionette becomes evidence of the paradox that ensues when we insist on a binary opposition between nature and culture or between feminine and masculine; and this is one reason why things are not so simple with her. Derrida argues that things are not simple with her because she displays the "equivocality of the living being" as both self-moving or spontaneous and moved by something other than itself, as both automotive and automatic. He concludes, "The living being is automotive, autonomous, absolutely spontaneous, sovereignly automotive, and at the same time perfectly programmed like an automatic reflex" (221). And it is the marionette as the double of the virgin girl—art as the double of nature—that shows us this paradox by displaying how "the phallic erection [that] comes to inhabit, haunt, and double that of the virgin girl. The virgin is inhabited by motion, movement, the essentially phallic law of the mario-nette" (221).

Derrida explains that the marionette is phallic not only because it is erect, hard and made of wood, and because it is operated like a machine or "hard-wired," but also because it is a substitute or actor that stands in (or up) for "the original," the effect of which it produces/reproduces. Someone else is pulling its strings, yanking its chain; and this reflexive action could be compared to the operations of phallic erection, which are not really in man's control. In the essay "Faith and Knowledge," Derrida describes the "phallic effect" as the effect of a marionette, both a dead machine and the symbol of fertility or life: "Is it not the colossal automaticity of the erection (the maximum of life to be kept unscathed, indemnified, immune and safe, sacrosanct), but also and precisely by virtue of its reflex character, that which is most mechanical, most separable from the life it represents? The phallic—is it not also, as distinct from the penis and once detached from the body, the marionette that is erected, exhibited, fetishized, and paraded in processions?" (2002a, 83).

Man's erection, like the marionette, is a double that simulates agency, a prosthesis of sovereignty. This prosthetic operation is the performance of sovereignty, erecting itself. The "facile comparison," as Derrida calls it, is not, however, the connection between phallic erection and the marionette that he finds most interesting. It is not just that the marionette participates in "the cult of the phallus," but rather that "the phallus is itself originally a marionette" (2009, 223). At this point, Derrida reminds the listener/reader that the word *phallos* "first designated in Greece and Rome for certain ceremonies, that simulacrum, that figured representation of an erect penis, hard, still rigid, precisely like a gigantic and artificially made-up puppet, made of tensed springs and exhibited during rituals and processions" (222). The phallus, originally the phallos, is a marionette, a "prosthetic representation of the penis in permanent erection" (222). Moreover, permanent erection, or "upping the ante" to the highest heights of majesty, the hyperbolic most of absolute sovereignty, is not possible for man (let alone woman), but only as a wooden woody or a fake phallus.

Insofar as the phallos is a prosthesis, it is "scarcely more masculine than feminine," "neither animal nor human" (2009, 222). And although it may not belong to the girl either, it "inhabits" or "haunts" her, not only because it too is a marionette, but also and moreover because it initiates her into the world of sexual difference, particularly at the moment when Derrida invokes Freud's essay "The Taboo of Virginity." Derrida mentions Freud's reference to Priapus's phallus in relation to a taboo on deflowering virgins that required "Indian young wives . . . to sacrifice their hymen on a wooden lingam (again a kind of marionette)," and among the Romans "the newly-wed wife at least has to sit on what Freud calls 'a gigantic stone phallus of

Priapus'" (223). Although Derrida does not discuss Freud's analysis of the fear of deflowering virgins, that account is relevant for deciphering the role of the girl in Derrida's seminar.

Aside from a general "dread" of women and fear of the sight of blood, Freud identifies two other main causes for the taboo of virginity, which he maintains continues into the present: the threat of castration and the threat of revenge through frigidity. In the first, along with the threat posed by the female sex as already castrated, there is the threat of her sex as castrating, which Freud describes as being "infected with her femininity." He diagnoses man's fear: "The man is afraid of being weakened by the woman, infected with her femininity and of then showing himself incapable. The effect coitus has of discharging tensions and causing flaccidity may be the prototype of what the man fears; and realization of the influence which the woman gains over him through sexual intercourse, the consideration she thereby forces from him, may justify the extension of this fear. In all this there is nothing obsolete, nothing which is not still alive among ourselves" ([1917], 198–99).

This passage signals a fear that femininity (which for Freud is associated with passivity) is contagious. Furthermore, the man in the postcoitus-weakened (feminine) position is flaccid, which seems to trigger fears of castration. Finally, Freud links this state to the woman's control over man, gained through sex. Also, the second fear of revenge through frigidity signals man's fear of woman's power over sex and that she could withhold it from him as a sort of punishment or revenge. Certainly, in either case, it seems that the man's fear is related to his sovereignty, or lack of it. He fears losing his sovereign power over the woman, even worse, becoming like her. When tied to the fear of deflowering virgins and the rituals surrounding that act, what Freud identifies as weakness, passivity, and powerlessness brought on by intercourse actually trigger fears of impotence. In other words, behind the fear of castration is the fear of impotence, the fear of loss of power, loss of sovereignty. The fear of deflowering virgins that is displaced onto the wooden phallos in the rituals described by Freud and mentioned by Derrida could be explained by the *fear of impotence*, and moreover by evidence of impotence discovered on the wedding night. Indeed, in some traditions, the sheets are examined for blood the morning after to make sure that the marriage was consummated (and perhaps that the woman was indeed a virgin). The ritualistic deflowering with a wooden phallos, however, destroys the evidence before the fact of the man's possible impotence on his wedding night. In this way, the man protects himself not against the threat of castration, or even the threat of revenge by his new bride, but rather from what Freud calls "showing himself incapable." It is noteworthy in this regard that the god Priapus may have a permanent erection, but he is also permanently impotent, which means that any deflowering only can be performed only by his phallos and not his phallus.

In addition to the fear of impotence, the man also seems to fear the girl's power, especially her power over him wielded in sex. This takes us back to Celan's "The Meridian" and the scene of the two girls turned to stone by a Medusa's head wielded now by the artist as an apotropaic against the power of those virginal girls engaged in innocent pleasures on their own, independent of man. So too it recalls Celan's opening invocation of Pygmalion, who is afraid of real girls and creates his beloved stone girl; because she is made of stone, she cannot reproduce. Does this fact signal a defect in the representation or reproduction of a girl? Or, rather might it signal another deeper fear on the part of man, a fear of women's powers of reproduction? Women's powers of reproduction take us beyond or between two marionettes, between nature and culture, between nature and art, as we have seen, all the more so today with so many assisted reproductive technologies. Again, man is trying to pull the strings of reproduction by controlling it through these technologies, including genetic engineering and cloning. Among so many other things, however, what Derrida's analysis of art and reproduction suggests is that man's supposed sovereignty over nature or culture is a performance, and one that he cannot keep up permanently.

Detumescence versus Castration

We could say that the fear of *girl power* and the fear of impotence, then, come to the same thing. For it is upon the girl's wooden phallos that man erects the fiction of his own virility. Like Medusa's head, she both reassures him by turning him to stone and threatens him with her power to do so. The reproduction of the permanent erection upon which the girl must sit to hide the evidence of man's potential impotence performs the fiction of his sovereign election to absolute phallic power. And yet, at the same time that this reproduction props up the fiction of his election to erection, it reveals both its own status as fake and empty of any real power. Think again of Priapus the impotent god of fertility, whose name has been given to the painful and dangerous medical condition priapism. This reflection leads Derrida to Aristotle's *The Parts of Animals*, where Aristotle wonders what would happen if an erection became permanent. Extending the Aristotelian line of thought on the issue of erection, Derrida provocatively concludes: "Perhaps tolerable for beasts and for demigods, this imperturbable and impassive erection would produce in men only impotence without the emission of semen, and thus without generative power, and would produce only pain without enjoyment. The pathology called priapism leads to death. And priapism is infinite ithyphallism, ithyphallism foreign to that detumescence that is the finitude of erection and that, as such, make possible the time of erection—which it threatens, of course, but to which it also gives its opportunity. A priapic, i.e., permanent and indefinite, erection is no longer even an erection—and it is a mortal pathology" (2009, 224–25). Aside from the comic effect of the ridiculous spectacle of permanent erection is the comedy of the spectacle of empty power, impotent power—that is, phallic power as such.

Derrida asks whether detumescence is castration. In other words, is flaccidity the same as castration? Freud at least suggests that the one leads to thoughts of the other. But Derrida prefers not to take on "this immense question frontally" (2009, 225). Rather, he takes another detour through Celan's "The Meridian" with its uncanny Medusa's head and marionettes. Another turn around the dance floor with his wooden leg. As at so many other times when Derrida insists that he will not approach his subject "frontally," here he says that he prefers to creep up on it "like a wolf, slowly, discreetly" (223). Although he advises his listeners (now readers) to undertake a systematic linear reading of Celan's speech, he takes a different route "because the actively interpretative, selective, and directed reading I am about to propose to you requires it" (225). This active interpretation is not a passive or flaccid interpretation that simply follows along from A to Z. Rather, its power, its uniqueness, "(a reading that to my knowledge has not yet been attempted)," requires its selectivity and electivity of passages that create the uncanny effect of an encounter, a unique encounter with what he calls "a certain poetic signature" that might allow us to see "where the poem is coming from and going—to free itself, by art, from art" (cf. 223; 227).

Following Derrida's turns, we discover that while there are moments when he addresses his subject frontally or fully erect, they don't last long. In another text, *The Animal that Therefore I Am*, he suggests that it is shameful to approach head-on, face-to-face, or standing upright: "There is a rhythmic difference between erection and detumescence. It is no doubt at the heart of what concerns us here, namely, a sentiment of shame related to standing upright—hence with respect to erection in general and not only phallic surrection—and to the face-to-face (2008, 36–37). Rather than approach frontally or head-on, the twists and turns through which he stages an encounter with where the poem is coming from and going—to free art from and by itself—operate according to a rhythm that presents something like an interpretation before the text as a type of foreplay. This happens literally when he creeps up on a passage that he eventually quotes in full, but only at the end of a session, as, after many, often dizzying revolutions, he allows the text to have the last word. But it also gives an interpretation—one possible among others, as he tells his audience/reader repeatedly—as a gift that makes us wait. The encounters that he stages through his interpretations before the texts are seemingly intended to announce the other with all of its uncanniness, for which we must wait. We must wait for the other to come. Derrida warns at the beginning of the seminar that he will make us wait. And, as usual, he does. And, as usual, it is worth the wait. But this exercise in waiting is also preparation for what he comes to call "the time of the other" through which "we" may hope to twist free of art by art and toward an encounter with what makes it uncanny. This is not just the deconstructive operation of revealing that the emperor has no clothes, that his majesty is the effect of smoke and mirrors, or that he is merely a puppet, a wooden woody. Through art as marionette, Derrida invokes, in the name of poetry (a "certain poetic signature"), something beyond it that moves us towards an encounter with the uncanny otherness of life itself. This otherness is not some-thing that can be manifest or reproduced. It is not the result of the virile insemination by some proper name whose authority exceeds all others. Rather, it is what Celan calls an "impossible path" and a "path of the impossible" (cf. 2009, 227). It cannot be conjured by the sovereign and his magic wand (or grand erection). Rather, it is a matter of chance, something that happens, an event, even an accident, for better or worse, that befalls us, or fells us with its own majesty, poetic majesty rather than sovereign majesty.

In what has become another technique of Derrida's deconstructive art, he uses one type of majesty to dethrone the other; in this case poetic majesty dethrones sovereign majesty.[8] Whereas sovereign majesty erects itself as the most, the grandest, the supreme, His Highness, poetic majesty opens onto an uncanny otherness that unseats any such self-certainty and deflates the illusion of sovereign erection. Whereas the performance of sovereignty claims to possess the power and potency of the "I can" that can master all others, the performance of poetry undoes the "I can" and renders it powerless and impotent. In some sense, what Derrida calls "the enigma of potency" begins in Heidegger when he demands that we "let beings be"; what does it mean to let beings be? What is this uncanny passive activity of letting be? This is a "row" that Derrida says he has been "hoeing here for years, namely that of a thought of the possible as im-possible, and the conditions of possibility as conditions of im-possibility. Or of im-potence." "But," he again stops himself. Just when he is getting to the point or bringing his analysis to a head, he says, "I will not continue frontally in this direction today" (2009, 259). He stops himself from addressing the issue head-on.

Poetic Majesty against Sovereign Majesty

Poetic majesty, or the majesty of poetry or art, is used against political majesty not only to show how political majesty is itself an art form, a performance or a fiction, but also to show a way out of the auto-affective and self-aggrandizing fable that presents itself as the Truth in order to terrorize all others to the point of death. Derrida describes this majesty against majesty:

> It is as if, after the poetic revolution that was reaffirming a poetic majesty
> beyond or outside political majesty, a second revolution, the one that takes
> one's breath away or turns one's breath in the encounter with the wholly other,
> came to try or to recognize, to try to recognize, or even—without cognizing or
> recognizing anything—to try to *think* a revolution in the revolution, a
> revolution in the very life of time, in the life of the living present. This discreet,
> even unobvious, even miniscule, even microscopic dethroning of majesty
> exceeds knowledge. Not to pay homage to some obscurantism of
> nonknowledge, but to prepare perhaps some poetic revolution in the political

revolution, and perhaps too some revolution in the knowledge of knowledge, precisely between the beast, the marionette, the head, the Medusa's head, and the head of His Majesty the sovereign. (2009, 273)

Derrida is describing a revolution in time that gives way to the time of the other, the time of the uncanny, the time of what unsettles our self-certainty. This does not mean merely displacing sovereignty from the self, the auto, to the other, or erecting the other as sovereign (cf. 245). Rather, poetic majesty opens the present, splits it, to reveal something other than phallic power at its heart. The beating heart of art and of life is not one automatic pumping machine or phallic organ but many forces and bodies tugging at one another such that we no longer know who or what is us/self or them/other.

It becomes clear that allowing time for the other is not giving it time to speak in a democratic debate; it is not setting aside an allotted time for a minority opinion. Neither is it making the other speak, nor speaking for the other. Rather, it is giving as letting. But again this is not merely a passive waiting. For, at bottom, Derrida's "giving the other its time" challenges the very distinction between active and passive, between power and impotence, virility and dissemination. This brings us back to his question of whether detumescence is the same as castration. Is impotence the same as powerlessness? Or, better yet, is the lack of erection the same as being cut off from any type of sovereignty, majesty, or agency? To think so, as Freud suggests, may be precisely to erect phallic power as the supreme form of sovereignty, that "certain sovereignty" that Derrida attempts to deconstruct in the name of another, namely a certain liberty: "The double bind is that we should deconstruct, both theoretically and practically, a *certain* political ontotheology of sovereignty without calling into question a certain thinking of liberty in the name of which we put this deconstruction to work" (2009, 301). Derrida says "a certain" to indicate that there are various forms of sovereignty, just as there are various forms of liberty and majesty; and he uses one against the other. Indeed, showing that there are various forms of sovereignty is the first step in dethroning that certain form that erects itself as the grandest, the most, the only, or we might say, the certain (to play on the English word that can mean either a specific one or certainty).

Derrida stages this encounter with the genesis of poetic majesty not by claiming that his interpretation is the grandest, the most, the only, the mother of all interpretations, but rather through what he calls elsewhere *dissemination* (cf. 1981). Dissemination, unlike the phallic erection of sovereignty that asserts its power over everything through its virile claims to know and control everything, spreads its seeds far and wide without producing a legitimate heir to the throne of phallic power. As we have seen, in other texts Derrida has used his concept of dissemination as a counterpoint to metaphors of inheritance and legitimacy that also sustain the fiction of a certain sovereign power as the right asserted through its might (cf. 1987). Dissemination, on the other hand, does not yield one truth or the right interpretation or the correct reading. Rather, by scattering proper names galore throughout *The Beast and the Sovereign*, Derrida's style of interpretation is one of cross-pollination and contamination with which he challenges claims to propriety, inheritance, and legitimacy.

As Derrida often reminds us, within the fiction of inheritance, legitimacy, and sovereignty, the girl is always illegitimate.[9] She cannot inherit the throne of His Majesty, the most, the highest, the erect and proper sovereign. Derrida asks, Can a woman hold this position of erection? And although within the traditional story she cannot, Derrida's seminar puts her smack in the middle of that story, that account of reason (or we might say logos of logos, playing with the double meaning of *logos* as both reason and account). She is, then, the reason for the sovereign's erection insofar as he sees her without being seen, and she goes about her business without a line in the dialogue; or the girls who watch as the Lion performs his right to everything; or Pygmalion's girl of stone who can neither speak nor reproduce, the wooden embodiment of man's ideal of feminine beauty, without any orifice from which to usher her own creations, be they words or offspring. The multiplication of girls behind the scenes of phallic power points to the ways in which the girl is an undecidable figure between nature and culture, animal and man, feminine and masculine. Yet she pulls the strings of the phallus at the same time that she is inhabited/haunted by it. In Derrida's *The Beast*, she performs the defloration that reveals the sovereign as also inhabited/haunted by impotence and that reveals his fabulous power as fable.

The figure of the innocent, graceful, spontaneous virgin girl is what erects the sovereign as the absolute authority, either over her directly (as in the story of Pygmalion or in La Fontaine's fable) or indirectly (as in Derrida's engagement with Celan's Büchner's *Lenz*). Girls are necessary witnesses to the fabulous Lion's declarations that might makes right. A girl is the Medusa's head that both reassures and threatens man by turning him to stone. She is the Medusa's head that is turned against the innocent girls, turning them into marionettes, and in so doing, redoubling the invocation of the figure of the girl. As such, she represents the paradox of representation, namely that any form of representation is a re-presentation that is as productive of its "original" as it is reflective. This paradox is what troubles Büchner's *Lenz* when he wants the Medusa's head to turn the beautiful innocent girls to stone exactly as they are in their pure and natural state, without changing and thereby contaminating them. Pygmalion thinks he can solve this problem by creating an ideal girl out of stone.

But Derrida's engagement with these moments makes clear that the ideal or virgin girl is already an artifice, a marionette. Yet things are still not so simple with this girl. She is not just one marionette among others but is between two marionettes, between the automobile that is nature and the automatic that is culture. She is neither a product of nature nor of culture but both/and. Her in-between or undecidable status makes her virginity always already contaminated (or inhabited/haunted) by the phallos. Like the Medusa's head, the virgin girl performs the paradoxical and double function of both reassuring man and threatening him, of propping up his erection even while exposing it as impotent. Her double role in the erection of phallic power reveals it as always merely a representative, a surrogate, a prosthesis, a wooden woody, that is erected on and through (likenesses, fables of) little girls, virginal statues who/that are subjected to the stick. In this way, slowly, creeping up, making us wait, Derrida hoists sovereign phallic power on its own petard by deconstructing its wooden platform, its artificial support, to reveal that it has been a fabulous fake, a phallos, all along.

Coda: Little Red Riding Hood and the Big Bad Wolf

In her essay "Devouring Figures: The Last Seminars of Jacques Derrida," Elizabeth Rottenberg begins with an anecdote about the difficulty of translating the word *gueule* as maw or as jaw. She asks, "Was it better to err on the side of the beast ('maw' being, according to the *OED*, 'the jaws or throat of a *voracious* animal') or was it better to err on the side of the idiom ('jaw' or 'jaws' translating more accurately the idiomatic quality of *gueule* in French)? Was it better to stress the voracity of the voracious, devouring mouth ('maw') or the linguistic performance of the talking, speaking mouth ('jaw') . . . ? Would there ever be a 'maw' in Little Red Riding Hood?" (Rottenberg 2011, 177).[10] Rottenberg goes on to analyze Derrida's references to Little Red Riding Hood in volume 1 of *The Beast and the Sovereign*, where he quotes Red Riding Hood twice: "Grandmother, what big teeth you have"; "Grandmother, what big ears you have." She argues that these two invocations of Little Red Riding Hood carry different aspects of orality and vociferation: the first calls attention to the mouth as the place of possible devouring; the second to the ears as listening to speech, which conjures the mouth as the place of speech (2011, 179). She concludes, "Thus orality has a double tongue, a double carry (*double portée*), and a double place" (179).

In the end, Rottenberg bears down on multiple meanings of carry or bear (*portée*) insofar as they call attention to the opposition between life and death, specifically bearing a child and bearing a death (perhaps of a child). Her analysis suggests that life and death, like the beast and the sovereign, cannot be separated. They are locked together in a double *portée* or double carry, carrying each other, one carried within the other. Life bears death and death bears life. She quotes Derrida on the double *portée* between birth and mourning: "At bottom, the true sense of the word 'porter' (*tragen, entragen*) is just as much determined by the carrying or bearing [*portée*] of life (the mother who carries her child) as it is by the carrying or bearing [*portée*] of death by life, of the dead by the living" (Rottenberg 2011, 181; brackets in original; cf. Derrida 2011, 153). Life and death, birth and mourning, locked together in the double carry of the verb *porter* in French or *bear* in English. The mother bearing her child . . . the mother burying her child. How do we bear it, the weight of this double burden, birth and mourning?

Rottenberg turns back to the fairy tale of Little Red Riding Hood, particularly the 1857 Grimm version, for a possible answer. Unlike in the 1697 Perrault version, which ends with the wolf eating Little Red Riding Hood, here a hunter rescues Little Red Riding from the belly of the wolf, and she has learned her lesson about trusting wolves. In her analysis of the story, Rottenberg sees this sequel as "fabulous," "not only because it brings the figure of the devouring wolf and the fantasm of devourment together, and not only because it rewrites death as life, but because translation, in this case, brings technology with it: namely, another set of jaws," the scissors used by the hunter to liberate—or we might say rebirth—Little Red Riding Hood and her grandmother (Rottenberg 2011, 181–82). "Death by devourment," concludes Rottenberg, "is rewritten as birth by cesarean"; or the death-bearing maw/jaw becomes the life-bearing belly (182). She provocatively suggests that translation as a figure for deconstruction is itself a form of carrying or bearing that uses technology—the scissors—to transform, transfer, carry us "from the *jaws that bite* to the *Jaws of Life*" (182). We could say that the cut of techne into physis is a form of rebirth that is necessary for birth itself. Little Red Riding Hood (and her grandma, or in Rottenberg's analysis, "grandmaw") is born out of the belly of the wolf. And in some sense, grandma/maw, Red Riding Hood, and the wolf are one and the same—or at least figures who assimilate one another.

In more recent feminist retellings of the story, the wolf is overcome by the grandma, the mother, or the daughter, Little Red Riding Hood herself, rather than by a man, the woodcutter. For example, Paula Rego's *Little Red Riding Hood Suite* (2003), which is comprised of seven images, shows Little Red Riding Hood's mother prodding the belly of the wolf (who is really a man) with a pitchfork and finally dressed in a wolf-fur-collared dress. And Kiki Smith's many works devoted to the Red Riding Hood theme challenge the fable of a man rescuing the girl and the old woman in various ways. For example, her print *Born* shows Little Red Riding Hood and Grandma emerging from the belly of the wolf on their own, as phoenix figures rising from the ashes. Her sculpture *Rapture* shows a full-grown, nude Red Riding Hood as a woman emerging from the belly of the wolf, suggesting that through the girl's encounter with the wolf, she becomes a woman (again without the help of the woodcutter). Discussing this work, Sarah Bonner says, "Rapture may represent the sexual woman released from the wolf's belly, or alternatively present the metamorphosis of the wolf into woman" (2012, 10). The fluidity between girl, woman, and wolf is prominent in two other works by Kiki Smith: *Gang and Girls and Pack of Wolves* (1999) and *Daughter* (1999). The first is composed of twelve painted-glass sheets displaying girls and wolves together, seemingly living in harmony. The second is a sculpture of a red-caped girl figure whose face is covered in fur, again suggesting that either the wolf has become a girl or vice versa, or perhaps that this hybrid "daughter" figure is the offspring resulting from the encounter between Little Red Riding Hood and the wolf. In all of her Little Red Riding Hood works, Smith calls into question the opposition between the girl and the wolf as fixed identifications. Rather, in her work, their identities are fluid; their identities are transformed or transferred— might we say carried—into each other.

The same might be said for our other woodsy girls roaming the forest—Hanna, Katniss, and Bella (and maybe even Sarah Palin and her daughters)—who use their wits and their bows to hunt and kill wild animals, whether rabbits and deer for survival, or big bad wolves—literal and figurative—who are hunting them. They are both hunters and hunted, girls and animals, natural innocents and killing machines. Like the goddess Artemis the huntress, they become figures for hunting, wild animals, wilderness, childbirth, and virginity. They become figures of rebirth from the artifice of techne, whether they wield a bow and arrow or a pair of scissors (or their knifelike equivalents). These virgin girls are naturals, that is, natural-born killers, trained by their fathers to hunt and survive, even if it means killing off their fathers in the process. As we have seen, caught between the machines of nature and culture, they both jam the gears and get the motor running.

Perhaps it is telling that in a 1998 advertisement for Chanel No. 5, the natural scent of Little Red Riding Hood (model Estella Warren) is not what announces her arrival to the fine-tuned nose of the wolf. Only when the perfumed supplement enhances her scent does this long-legged, big-breasted Little Red both attract and tame the wolf. This sexy, silky, high-heeled Red Riding Hood turns to face the wolf that pursues her, puts her finger to her lips to say "shhh," both teasing and lulling the beast, then bounces out the door, leaving the hungry wolf to throw back his head and howl with desire.

FOUR

Rearview Mirror: Art, Violence, and Sublimation

> Athena invented the rear-view mirror, which allows us to face the horror,
> not face to face, but beginning from the duplicate, the simulacrum.
>
> —JULIA KRISTEVA, *The Severed Head*

If we interpret deconstruction as a form of translation as transference, we
have moved into the territory of psychoanalysis. Indeed, if poetic majesty
acts to unseat sovereign majesty through the cut that carries with it rebirth,
as in the story of Little Red Riding Hood, then psychoanalysis may be
the discourse best equipped for articulating the dynamics of this wound
that is also a source of life. In other words, psychoanalysis may provide the
tools with which to analyze the thorny relationship between violence and
life, particularly through the concepts of death drive and sublimation.
Returning to our violent girls, hunting and hunted, deconstruction does
more than merely suggest a role reversal, that Little Red Riding Hood kills
and devours the wolf. Bloodthirsty girls may provide good entertainment,
and they may be even a step up from bloodthirsty wolves, but we are still
left with bloodshed and violence. But how might the scissors that cut—what
psychoanalysis calls the operation of castration—lead to rebirth or renewal

beyond violence? Can representations of the cut or the wound, that is to say violence, sublimate violence and take us beyond both individual and political sovereignty? How is it that poetic majesty works as an antidote to sovereign majesty and thereby quells its violence?

Do representations of violence incite or quell violent desires and actions? This question—the question of the relation between mimesis and catharsis—is as old as Western philosophy itself. In this chapter, I turn to Julia Kristeva to begin to answer these questions. Using Kristeva's latest work on the dynamics of sadomasochistic subjectivity and sublimation through art, I describe some of the differences between representations of violence that perpetuate violent desires and actions, and representations of violence that sublimate violent desires and thereby prevent violent actions. To my knowledge, Kristeva never gives a sustained and straightforward answer to this question. Indeed, her many discussions of language, representation, and visual arts, along with theatre, dance, poetry, music, and installation pieces, suggest that artistic representation and certain kinds of signifying practices are sublimatory, that they can become productive homes—if only temporarily—for aggressive drives. Yet exactly how and why some representations sublimate violence and others stimulate it is not so clearly delineated. This distinction becomes especially vexed when Kristeva, in works such as *New Maladies of the Soul* and *The Sense and Non-Sense of Revolt*, criticizes the society of the spectacle. In these works she argues that media spectacles flatten psychic space and threaten to kill off the psyche or soul once and for all. This leads me to ask: What distinguishes representation as spectacle from representation as sublimation, or as transformation?

In more psychoanalytic terms, the question is: What distinguishes forms of representation that work through the sadomasochistic drives that inaugurate our entrance into language and society, from forms of representation that participate in acting out those aggressive instincts? My attempt to answer these questions will focus on two rarely discussed but to my mind pivotal texts in Kristeva's corpus: the 1998 catalogue she created to accompany the exhibit of decapitated heads that she curated at the Louvre, entitled *Visions capitales* (recently translated [2012] for an English-speaking audience with the more graphic and spectacular title *The Severed Head: Capital Visions*), and a talk that she gave at Columbia University in 2006 at the Dead Father Symposium, entitled "A Father is Being Beaten to Death," which is reflected in parts of her books *This Incredible Need to Believe* (2009; first published in Italian, 2006) and *Hatred and Forgiveness* (2010; first published in French, 2005), written around that same time.

A Father Is Being Eaten: Retelling the Tale of the Primal Horde

In part, both *The Severed Head* and "A Father is Being Beaten" are Kristeva's reworking of Freud's *Totem and Taboo*, particularly in relation to the sadomasochistic origins of subjectivity and signification. Kristeva puts sadomasochistic violence at the heart of signification itself, which for her can be a safeguard against violent acting out, but only if it doesn't become a new form of fundamentalism in the name of which we act out our most violent fantasies on the bodies of others. I will argue that it is the precarious and interminable process of working through our sadomasochistic origins that determines whether or not we represent or act out, and whether or not our representations transform our violent impulses or merely feed them.

Since at least the writing of *Powers of Horror* (1982), Kristeva has repeatedly returned to Freud's *Totem and Taboo* in order to retell the story of the primal horde, which not only inaugurates civil society with its taboos against murder and incest, but also inaugurates representation in all of its forms. This is a story of the violent origins of the primary processes of condensation and displacement that make signification possible and brand us as human beings. In a sense, it is Freud's answer to the most primal, yet most profound, of questions: Where do we come from? In Kristeva's retelling of the story of the origins of the speaking subject, Freud's murdered father becomes the beaten father, while Freud's forbidden mother becomes the beheaded mother. The father beaten to death and the beheaded mother not only inaugurate the prohibitions against murder and incest, as the Freudian story goes, but also open up the possibility of sublimating the violence necessary to become speaking subjects—a sadomasochistic violence that Kristeva insists is still necessary on both the individual and the social levels. To set the stage for Kristeva's latest revisions of the Freudian origin story, which revolves around the beaten father and the beheaded mother, I will sketch some of her earlier engagements with *Totem and Taboo*, in *The Sense and Non-Sense of Revolt*, and before that in *Powers of Horror*.

As we know, Freud gives a provocative explanation for the origins of the processes of idealization and sublimation that initiate religion, civil society, and representation. This is a story of the body giving way to the law, and of the animal giving way to humanity. His story is familiar to us: what he calls a "band of brothers" kill and eat a "man" Freud calls their "father" and afterwards totemize the father out of guilt; they then develop prohibitions against murder and incest in order to prevent any one of the brothers from meeting the fate of the father. On this account, there was one superior male (the father) who hoarded the females and shunned the other males (the sons or brothers). Individually none of the other males could over-power the superior male, but one day they banded together to kill him and assimilate his power through their cannibalistic feast. At this point, they are not much different from a pack of wolves ripping into the alpha male. What distinguishes them from wolves, however, is that they subsequently *idealize* their "prey," the superior father, to the point that "[t]he dead father became stronger than the living one had been" (Freud [1913], 501). Thus, they not only assimilate his power but also restrict that power through internalized prohibitions or laws, resulting both from their guilt and from their submission to the ideal or symbolic father who now replaces the real one.

In *Powers of Horror*, Kristeva's most significant revision of the Freudian narrative is her insistence on the primary role of the maternal body in the cannibalistic, and subsequent ritualistic, meal. Here it is the primal feast that fascinates Kristeva. And along with the prohibitions against murder and incest, she focuses on the prohibition against cannibalism at the dawn of humanity. This concern leads her to an analysis of food prohibitions in general, which she maintains always take us back to the maternal body, the first source of nourishment and the first source of frustration, pleasure become anguish. Or, in the terms of Melanie Klein, the good breast becomes the bad breast, an ambivalence that Kristeva attempts to capture with her notion of the abject, which signifies what is both fascinating and horrifying.

Like Freud, Kristeva bases her analysis on anthropological literature, particularly Mary Douglas's study of filth and defilement. She suggests that fear of the generative power of the mother makes her body abject and inedible, and thereby makes all bodies abject and inedible: "I give up cannibalism because abjection (of the mother) leads me toward respect for the body of the other, my fellow man, my brother" (1982, 79; parentheses in the original). Through the ambivalent struggle with the maternal body and the incest taboo, all human bodies become inedible.

On the level of the individual, an oral aggression related to both food and speech revolves around a fear of loss of the mother aggravated by threats of punishment by the father (1982, 39). The child feels aggression in response to its fear both of the loss of maternal satisfaction and of paternal prohibition instituted by the incest taboo. Kristeva sees a pre-objectal aggression that comes from bodily drives and latches onto totemic symbols that stand in for, rather than represent, everything threatening and scary in the child's young life: "Fear and the aggressivity intended to protect me from some not yet localizable cause are projected and come back to me from the outside: 'I am threatened'" (39). The child responds to both deprivation and prohibition with aggressive impulses, which in the case of the maternal body may literally include the urge to bite or devour, to incorporate, the maternal body in order to hold on to it (cf. 39).

The child's own aggressivity, then, is projected onto something outside of itself, for example a phobic animal, as a shield not only against the deprivation and prohibition exercised toward it by its parents but also against its own violent impulses. At this stage, these impulses revolve around incorporation as an attempt to devour and thereby possess the parental love (not-yet) object. At the same time that the child is learning language and incorporating the words of its parents, it is trying to incorporate the parents themselves. For the infant, the mouth is the first center of bodily cathexis associated with pleasure, deprivation, and language acquisition. Words, along with breast milk and food, pass through the infant's mouth. Kristeva interprets the phobic's fantasies of being bitten, eaten, or devoured by a scary animal as a projection of his or her own aggressive drives, particularly the urge to bite, eat, or devour the maternal body. As we will see, in "The Severed Head" the mother's face becomes the quintessential figure for the condensation of the abject, with its scary, devouring mouth and radiant, reassuring, loving smile.

In *The Sense and Non-Sense of Revolt*, Kristeva reads Freud's *Totem and Taboo* in terms of various forms of assimilation: the assimilation of authority through cannibalism, the assimilation of the body, and of representation, and the assimilation of language. But now she adds an emphasis on the break between the timelessness of animal instincts linked to bodily drives and the linear temporality of signification onto, and into, which they are discharged. She suggests that the institution of memory in the totemic rituals represses timelessness, the timelessness of the drives. Her invocation of archaic timelessness gives us another motive for the repetition of rituals that assimilate the authority and power of the primal father. Rather than just repeating the crime as a reminder of lack and debt on the one hand, and of the mobility of power on the other, repeating the timelessness of animal-experience-become-bodily-drive also frees us from prohibition and guilt and puts us in touch with the rhythms of the body and its pleasures and pains outside of linear time. Rather than merely repeat guilt and prohibition, idealization opens the space for a repetition of timelessness within linear time, a repetition that Kristeva identifies with the celebratory excess, or jouissance, of the feast. The origin story is not just the story of fixed totems or taboos, but also the story of how bodily drives become meaningful through signifying rituals even as they exceed those rituals. It is the story of animal instincts become human drives; ultimately it is the story of the fluidity of desire.

Desire is not conceived of as the flip side of prohibition; rather, desire reverberates with longing for an archaic timelessness of our embodiment. On the level of the social, this timelessness is associated with animality and with the transition from animal to human, while on the level of the individual, it is associated with the infant's relation to the maternal body and with the transition from dependence to independence. In a sense, this timelessness is the absolute unity of being and meaning—what Freud might call the death drive, and later what Kristeva associates with the timelessness of death itself, which is outside of time and invisible, but can be rendered visible through artistic representation: "Death exists outside time: we can't see it; we must be content with varying our capital visions of it. Absolute cult or ultimate revenge?" (2012, 123).

The Malady of Ideality

I will return to this question, but for now we can describe sublimation not only as a process of redirecting sexual and aggressive instincts à la Freud's totem and taboo, but also as a process of discharging the timelessness of the drives (of the animal and of the preoedipal subject) into time (the temporality of the human and of the individual). Indeed, as I have argued elsewhere, we can go further and diagnose Freud's account of the killing-become-murder and subsequent guilt-become-prohibition as a displacement of this archaic timelessness into taboos—"Thou Shalt Not"—that take the form of universal principles, eternal truths, or divine (timeless) commandments (see Oliver 2004). This operation is the displacement of the timelessness of bodily drives into the eternal through which absolute good becomes an unforgiving ideal opposed to its abject opposite, absolute evil. The ideals of Good and Evil are beyond the realm of our embodied finite animality, and thereby deny everything bodily and finite in life—which, of course, is the process that Freud describes in *Totem and Taboo* as the violent beginnings of religion.

In terms of psychoanalysis, this form of idealization becomes a harsh and punishing superego that makes extreme demands as a defense against contamination by its disowned and abjected otherness, which it must exclude to define itself as clean and proper. Kristeva associates this form of idealization and abjection with fundamentalism and the self-righteous violence to which it can lead. She says, "The pure and absolute subject—call him the purifier—defends himself against the maternal from which he is separating through anti-taint rituals while at the same time defending himself against the murder of the father through feelings of guilt, contrition, repentance. Therefore what appears to be purity in the eyes of the religion and the purifiers is only an obsessional surface that conceals a veritable architecture of purity"; and "[T]o fight the various forms of fundamentalism and violence that appear to be the sorry privilege of this end of the century," we need to take "into consideration what produces it, namely, the disgust with taint and the consequent contrition, repentance, and guilt that present themselves as qualities of religion but also profoundly constitute the psychical life of the being capable of symbolicity: the speaking being" (2000, 22). In *This Incredible Need to Believe*, she calls this type of religious idealization that leads to violence the "malady of ideality" (2009, 18, 23).

We have now come full circle, back to a more nuanced version of the question with which we started: namely, What determines whether repetitions of the primal festival will take the form of violent acting out or sublimation of violence? Can we determine what rituals or signifying practices discharge the sadomasochistic drives at the heart of subjectivity by inflicting violence on others, and what rituals sublimate those drives and thereby transform the desire for violence and death into something creative? Within Kristeva's terminology, another version of our question is, What distinguishes perversion from sublimation? Certainly the answer to this question has everything to do with the processes of idealization and representation that Freud describes in *Totem and Taboo,* and that Kristeva elaborates throughout her work as the move from animal to human on the social level, and on the individual level, the move away from the maternal body and towards the paternal law—what in everyday language we call *weaning.*

A Mother Is Being Beheaded

Tracing our fascination with decapitation, beheading, and severed heads from prehistoric cave paintings through Andy Warhol's Marilyn Monroe diptych, in *The Severed Head* Kristeva repeatedly argues that all of these detached heads represent both the mother's face—that primal lost loving gaze—and representation itself, insofar as we associate thought with the head. The figure of the head brings together our most archaic fears and desires along with our most effective means for sublimating them. Kristeva's focus on the head, particularly in relation to the guillotine, prefigures Derrida's concern with the death penalty in his seminar conducted the very year after she curated the *Visions capitale* exhibit at the Louvre, and his later emphasis on the head as capital in *The Beast and the Sovereign.* There, he asks if perhaps the *bêtise* that he has been discussing in relation to divide between man as sovereign and animal as beast is not proper to man after all, but rather is proper to all living beings, or at least all beings with heads, all "capital beings" (Derrida 2009, 192). That is, all beings with heads (and central nervous systems and faces, mouths, eyes, etc.) may be capable of sovereignty and therefore of stupidity. Derrida also associates the head or capital vision with standing above and looking down on everything else as the sovereign. He pokes fun at philosophers who think that man's erect posture separates him from other animals and makes him sovereign over them. And certainly the connection between man's erect posture and man's erect organ is not lost on Derrida (cf. 2009, 201–02). Indeed, there are two heads here, not always acting as one. As we will see, Kristeva too makes this association between the head and the phallus, and therefore between decapitation and castration.

In *The Severed Head*, relating early cannibalistic rituals and skull fetishes to Freud's narrative of the primal horde, Kristeva once again transfers the originary founding violence from Freud's paternal figure to a maternal one. She claims that "the skull and the face, primary targets for the gaze, appear to us as privileged stations in the loss of maternal dependence. To assimilate the head of the other, to absorb the mother's milk of the brain . . . the cannibalistic ritual is as much if not more an appropriation of the mother's power than a devouring of the father-tyrant. . . . Thus we may read in [the totemic feast] a double celebration: that of the rival phallic father and that of the mother who abandoned us. . . . From this totemic perspective, the assimilation of the head also seems to be a possible archaic equivalent for incest" (2012, 16–17). Indeed, she calls the phallic cover up of maternal power a "construction 'after the fact' (Nächtraglich)" (82). Thus, she concludes: "To eat, to kill, to possess, to represent" (17).

On both the social and individual levels, we become speaking subjects by moving away from literal killing and eating and towards their metaphorical analogues in representation, assimilation, and substitution. Rather than eat the primal father or the mother's milk, we assimilate their words; and rather than kill them, we substitute symbols for our violent impulses, for example, images of severed heads. Yet Kristeva insists that these representations are sublimatory only insofar as they do not merely represent aggressive drives but rather discharge them, and more importantly, transform them. In *The Severed Head*, she uses such words as *alchemy, transubstantiation, transformation, transfiguration, passage, modulation, osmosis, metabolization, compensation,* and at the extreme, *resurrection, salvation,* and *rebirth,* to describe the process by which representation sublimates bodily drives, particularly primal urges for cannibalism, incest, and murder.

As she does when describing the revolution in poetic language in her early work, she insists that the intimate revolt, as she now calls it, which she associates with becoming an individual and that is repeated in each sublimatory representation, is not mimesis or a copying of drives in language (2012, 50–51). Bodily drives are neither the objects represented nor the referents of those objects (or images or symbols, as the case may be). Rather, a sign replaces the absent body (which always takes us back to the absent maternal body) through an *imprint*, an *infiltration*, an *inscription* of the body. The missing body, and at some level any missing object, including the phallus threatened with castration, is always the mother's missing face, source of joy and terror. Kristeva claims that we hallucinate her, see her image, and then fabricate word-signs. We thereby compensate for our separation from her, the cut, by taking control through representation: "For capital disappearance of mother's face, I substitute capital vision— images words language," which is another form of "incarnation" (5–6).

As always, Kristeva emphasizes the materiality of representation—in the case of severed heads, drawing, painting, and sculpture. Through art, we can get distance from our wounds and give them meaning that allows us to work through trauma and protects us from the worst violence: "No bombast, no savagery, you are distanced and sheltered from the cannibals, the terrorists" (2012, 86). Through art, she says, "slaughter turned to image assuages the violence, more or less repressed or mastered, of individuals and nations" through "alchemy in which the representation comes of a grieving, a renunciation, a castration, a death. There is something beyond death, the artistic experience says, there is resurrection. . . . Decapitation is a privileged space." (75–76). The idea is that rather than decapitate, we draw or paint severed heads.

Kristeva goes so far as to say that these visions of severed heads are the opposite of acts of decapitation. Discussing the French Revolution and the Reign of Terror, she begins a chapter on the guillotine: "In opposition to the imaginary intimacy with death, which transforms melancholy or desire into representation and thought, lies the rational realization of the capital act. Vision and action are polar opposites here, and the revolutionary Terror confronts us with that revolting abjection practiced by humanity under the guise of an egalitarian institution of decapitation" (2012, 91). She concludes the chapter, "[T]he profusion of images and symbols has a chance of thwarting the temptations of real actions. . . . After all, if art is transfiguration, it has political consequences" (101–02).

At this point, it seems as if Kristeva answers our original question with a resounding affirmation, namely, that representations quell rather than incite violence; indeed, representations may be the only way to prevent the worst violence. And, although the question of whether all representation prevents violence is still an open one, we have begun to get some clues as to how representation sublimates violent drives. First and foremost, representation transforms drives into something else, words, painting, sculpture, through which they are discharged without resorting to violence. Second, representation takes the place of the missing maternal face and thereby compensates for the absence and loss that incite violence, and also thereby softens and counterbalances the paternal prohibitions against cannibalism, murder, and incest, that allow us to live together. Third, art— and we could add psychoanalysis—allows us to distance ourselves from the loss and pain, and this detachment protects us from their crippling effects.

In *Hatred and Forgiveness*, Kristeva likens this detachment to a mother's love for a child that she must let go; there, she calls this process *de-passion*, or *de-passioning*, which is also a de-eroticizing necessary for sublimation of sadomasochistic drives that simultaneously threaten and inaugurate speech. In addition, artistic representation transforms the artist from a passive victim of trauma into an active agent of creativity. Thus, art transforms its subjects, in both senses of the word *subject*, the subject matter of the work and the creator of the work (see 2012, 63).

The relationship between the work of art and working through trauma takes us to our second, and more difficult, question: What sorts of representations prevent violence and what sorts actually incite violence? Certainly we have seen enough inflammatory rhetoric, particularly from religious fundamentalists of all sorts, to know that not all representation quells violence; rather, some exhorts it. Kristeva begins to answer this question in *The Severed Head* when she suggests that in order to be sublimatory, representation has to avoid becoming dogmatic, ideological, or fundamentalist. Conversely, when representation becomes dogmatic or ideological, it risks perpetuating rather than preventing violence. Indeed, it can become the ideal in the name of which we commit violent acts.

So, how do we avoid becoming dogmatic and ideological? Kristeva answers that when "[t]he passage becomes permanent, the thinking and risk that initially guided the line insidiously take shelter in perversion, dogmatism, marginalist ideology. . . . How to escape it? Quite simply through talent that does not succumb to the object, that avoids the fetish . . . through the invention of an unprecedented form, which doesn't shrink from abjection but reshapes our vision so that we see it with new eyes" (2012, 108). The object of art cannot become a fetish; rather it must always be a passage, a transition, and fluid rather than fixed. We must concentrate on the work of art, in its double meaning, rather than the artwork as an object. It is the process of figuration, particularly the drive force or primary processes that motivate it, that make art sublimatory, not the object of art per se. This is why one and the same art work or art object can aggravate or alleviate violence. And this is why Kristeva insists that we must maintain persistent "faithfulness to the cut," which simultaneously does both. We must leave open the wound, the trauma or loss, the horror, out of which creative representation is born, and through which it offers us rebirth, as she would say (108). Faithfulness to the cut that offers a rebirth recalls Elizabeth Rottenberg's interpretation of deconstruction as translation, as transference through the cut, illustrated in the story of Little Red Riding reborn from the belly of the wolf thanks to the woodcutter's scissors.

The difference, then, between spectacles that incite violence and art that sublimates it is that spectacles reinforce one way of seeing the world, while works of art open up new ways of seeing; they are an "antimetaphysical metaphysics," which constantly questions the foundations of all fundamentalisms: "abandon the spectacle and find a kind of face that has not yet found its face, that never will, but that never stops seeking a thousand and one ways of seeing. This is the intimacy they make us imagine, sensual seekers of the visible incarnation, the path of incarnation" (2012, 127). The process that Kristeva describes is an ongoing one of cathexis and de-cathexis that leads to more questions than answers. For without constant questioning, any interpretation or belief risks becoming fetishized fundamentalism, in the name of which we kill and "eat" each other.

A Father Is Being Beaten

In the essay "A Father Is Being Beaten to Death," as well as in *This Incredible Need to Believe*, Kristeva continues to delineate the difference between opening up questioning and closing it down. In "A Father" she describes her analysis of the child's identification with a beaten and suffering father as a rereading of Freud's *Totem and Taboo*, inflected by his theories in "A Child Is Being Beaten," where the guilt that underlies the being-beaten fantasy is the underside of desire for the father. Following Freud, she argues that the being-beaten fantasy is at the origin of individuation and subject constitution, and of sexual difference, now described in terms of differential relations to the beaten fantasy. If, in *The Severed Head*, sadomasochism is what Kristeva calls "the secret of the unconscious," here sadomasochism takes center stage as the flip side of sublimation. Language is both derived from, and sublimates, sadomasochistic desires for incest and murder of both parents, as well as the superego's pleasure in self-punishment for those very desires. Both the desires and their prohibitions are simultaneously channeled into representation. This, of course, is the familiar story of Freud's totem and taboo.

The guilt in killing the primal father comes from identification with him and his suffering, which is an essential part of the dynamic of substitution initiated by totemic rituals. In order for a symbol to substitute for the dead father, the son (or daughter) must first be able to identify with him and his suffering. And for Kristeva, the first substitution for the mother as object of incestuous desire is a narcissistic one wherein the infant's own body takes the place of the missing maternal body, through autoeroticism. But in order for the next stage in the process of substitutions to take place, the intensity of the eroticism connected to sadomasochistic desires for both parents must be transferred to language. Representation itself becomes a new love object that enables us to survive the loss of the maternal body and skirt the punishment of the paternal law (Kristeva 2006). We could simply say that through representation we cope with all loss, guilt, and punishment, whether the traumatic loss of the mother's face and our infantile connections to our first caregivers, or the big and small losses and victimizations that we suffer throughout our lives. Indeed, in order to survive them, we must take pleasure, even if perverse pleasure, in representing our melancholy experiences. Kristeva postulates, "In addition to *masochistic perversity* ('I take pleasure in the fantasy of being beaten') is the *sublimatory jouissance* of my own capacity to say and to think *for and with* the beloved/loving. I want to emphasize that from the beginning sublimation accompanies this perverse defense, and perversion acts as sublimation's double" (2006, 4; emphases in original).

The sadomasochistic identification with the beaten father is a defense against the father of the law and his punishment and thereby an essential part of the process of idealization that enables the intimate revolts necessary for individuation. The suffering father is the latest incarnation of Kristeva's imaginary father, introduced in *Tales of Love* as the necessary support for the move away from the maternal body and towards the paternal law.

Here, the suffering father plays the role of bridge between the two. His incarnation and victimization allow the subject to bond with a paternal most like itself; helpless, the infant or child as victim of the paternal law can find an alternate ideal in the father as victim. This identification supports the intimate revolt against the paternal authority that, in a paradoxical move, authorizes the subject and its entrance into the symbolic.

An identification with the beaten father counterbalances the punishing paternal super-ego by allowing the girl or boy sadomasochistic pleasure in punishment, which is doubled by sadistically turning the tables on the punishing father of the law and subjecting him to a beating, and then in turn masochistically identifying with his victimhood and what becomes sweet suffering. Kristeva says, "Beaten, I join my father once again; we are united by these nuptials under the whip. . . . 'We are both in love, and guilty, we both deserve to be beaten'" (2006, 5, 6). The passion of Christ is Kristeva's prime example of the "a father is being beaten to death" fantasy. Substituting the Christian fantasy of the suffering Christ beaten to death for the Freudian father murdered and eaten by the primal horde, Kristeva goes on to describe how identification with him supports the possibility of sublimation and the transfer of erotic intensity to symbolic activity itself:

> The resexualization of the ideal father as Man of Passion brings about an unprecedented *resexualization of representation itself*, of the very activity of fantasizing and of speaking. . . . The activity of representing-speaking-thinking, attributed to the father in patrilineal societies and which connects me to him, now becomes the privileged realm of sadomasochistic pleasure, the "kingdom" indeed, where suffering opens out, justifies and appeases itself. . . . *Perversion and sublimation are the flip sides of this flexibility, if not of this fabulous suspension of the incest taboo induced by the beaten-to-death father.* (2006, 7; emphases in original)

Again, Kristeva emphasizes incestuous desires and their taboos as the primary motivators for becoming speaking subjects. Representation not only compensates for the loss of these first loves, but also transforms desire for them into desire for language. Moreover, it transforms the passive victim of parental love and punishment into an active agent, while also turning the threatening parents into passive victims. The punishing father becomes the beaten father and the castrating mother becomes the beheaded mother. The perpetrator becomes the victim—but one with whom we identify; and with these sadomasochistic fantasies we find both revenge and reunion through imaginary and symbolic satisfactions. In this way, we not only separate from our parents to become individuals, but also we cope with the pain of that separation, the separation that prefigures all others.

But Kristeva also insists that imaginary and symbolic identification with suffering is a depassioning; so it is at once the transfer of erotic drives into representation and the transformation of those drives from passion to depassion, from eroticism to de-eroticism. And it is this transformation that allows us to embrace them, that puts them beyond the taboo, and provides us with sublimatory jouissance. Ultimately, with and against the death drive, representation makes the primary separation—which comes to stand for all pain, loss, trauma, and the very meaninglessness of life—into something meaningful, even sacred. Kristeva says, "understood as a traversal, by thought, of the unthinkable: of nothingness, uselessness, the vain and the mad," we are confronted not with religion but with the sacred (2006, 8).

This distinction between religion and the sacred brings us back to the fragile distinction between dogmatism and sublimation. When the sacred becomes fixed in religion, it becomes dogmatic and risks becoming fundamentalism through which we justify violence. It becomes the malady of ideality. But if the process of idealization necessary for a meaningful life is held open to constant questioning and reinterpretation through new forms of representation, then there is the possibility for sublimation of the sadomasochistic drives, which might prevent such violence. Rather than latching on to the ideal and becoming fanatical about it, we open it up to new ways of seeing, new fantasies of death and rebirth.

This is what Kristeva does in her own work, signaled by her use of questions that provide different ways of interpreting the same phenomena. For example, in *The Severed Head*, she asks, "What is the power of representation? Does the image succumb to the violence of death, or does it possess the gift of modulating it?" (2012, 10). This style of constant back-and-forthing, of either/or, of both/and, is also what sometimes makes her work frustrating and difficult to pin down. But also it is what opens it up to interpretation. Through the use of questions throughout her writing, she leaves open possibilities and complexities rather than closing them down or resolving them.

Kristeva maintains that the challenge to continually question our own investments in violence is unique to psychoanalysis. In her introduction to

This Incredible Need to Believe, entitled "The Big Question Mark," she argues that speaking in analysis becomes a questioning that "renders us capable of new bonds . . . the bond of investment in the process of symbolization itself" (2009, xv). With its constant reinterpretations of our losses and frustrations, it allows us to take pleasure in the pain of separation and of reunion over and over again in language. "The founder of psychoanalysis," she says, "began by making love lie down on the couch. In order to return to the love of the father and the mother, and on taking the gamble . . . that 'I' am capable of going beyond my genitors indeed beyond myself and my loves, on the condition of being subject to perpetual dissolution in analysis, in transference and counter-transference. This presupposes that there is not only a Dead Father, but also figures of paternity and of loves, in the plural, in which I take pleasure, which I kill and which I resuscitate when I speak, love and think" (2006, 11). Even more than art, psychoanalysis allows us to kill and resuscitate in speech as protection against the pain and suffering caused by our violent drives.

Medusa's Head

Like Athena protected by (and from) Medusa's head, psychoanalysis provides a rearview mirror in which we can see ourselves reflected over and over again in new ways. By so doing, with and against religion and its too often deadly call for violence, psychoanalysis opens up the sacred space of intimate revolt, which Kristeva calls psychic space or the life of the mind, or we could say, thought itself. Psychoanalysis acts as a counterbalance to the deadly force of fundamentalisms by offering "a space for reflection in which the effort of clarification takes precedence over the deadly confrontation between a tendency for regression on the one hand and the explosion of the death drives on the other, which together now threaten our globalized humanity" (2006, 11). This is possible because of the self-reflexivity symbolized by Medusa's gaze and the threat to mimesis that it poses. In other words, Medusa's gaze is reflected back on her, and it is her own deadly power that immobilizes her and counteracts her deadly effects. Yet this operation does not take place through the mere representation of her gaze or her power. Rather, the ricochet of her gaze, like the deconstructive jujitsu that turns a force back on itself, uses mimesis to destroy the illusion of the sovereign truth of representation, or the representation of sovereignty as the invocation of its own power.

In the words of Louis Marin, "The head of Medusa, then, is the defensive and offensive weapon wielded by wisdom in its war against the passions" (1990, 139). Perseus slays Medusa by keeping his distance and turning the Gorgon's own power against her by substituting her gaze for his own—she is forced to look at herself (cf. Marin 1990, 143). Discussing Caravaggio's painting "Head of Medusa," Marin argues, "for Caravaggio's painting not only makes representation visible in what is represented but also uses mimesis to destroy the mimetic process" (2000, 141). As we have seen, Kristeva also insists that the Medusa effect is not one of mimesis or representation. Rather, she argues that the power of the Medusa and other images of severed heads—perhaps art in general—is one of transformation and transference. It is not that art reflects reality or represents it, but rather that it transforms it, and through art we can transfer our desires and fears into socially acceptable containers, so to speak, without acting out our violent fantasies.

For Marin, the Medusa effect turns representation back on itself in a way that reflects its own reflective operations as part of a process that creates the effect of truth, and by so doing undermines that very effect: "The parodic process of displacement repeats the very operation in which painting destroys itself: the parody mimics itself, as it designates its own operation of collapse and thereby avoids any claim to embody the truth" (1990, 137). Through displacement, art transforms that which it "looks at" by showing that the gaze itself is transformative and thereby undermines any notion of absolute truth. Returning to the Kristevan framework, we could say that art is an antidote to fundamentalisms insofar as it reveals that there is no such thing as seeing things in themselves as they are in reality, because all looking always already involves operations of displacement and projection. The flip side of what could be the depressing fact, if you will, that all looking is projection, is that certain kinds of "looking"—artistic, creative, and poetic varieties—can be transformative.

In this way, art becomes an antidote to Reason with a capital *R*, in whose name we commit all sorts of atrocities. In Derrida's terms, artistic majesty or poetic majesty can unseat sovereign majesty's reasons—reason in the sense of rationality, and reason in the sense of justification or excuse. Discussing Medusa, Marin puts it:

> The representation of Medusa's gaze in the reflecting and reflexive mirror is a ruse and a machination. An element of reason—prospect—reversed or overturned, results in the reflection and retaliation of reason. The gaze is trapped by the eye in confrontation between weakness and strength, life and death. The painting is, first of all, Medusa petrifying herself with her own gaze in the present and immediate moment of polemical violence, before assuming a place of power on the breast of Jupiter's daughter as an attribute of the latter's divine institution. (1990, 143)

The round bronze eye of Perseus's shield stands in for his own as the technological supplement that at once protects him from the truth and renders it impotent.

Medusa's likeness on the shield of Athena performs a similar double operation. Recall that according to Freud the image of Medusa both threatens castration and reassures man of his virility by scaring him stiff. As usual, Kristeva complicates the Freudian interpretation by making Medusa into a figure of abjection and ambivalence associated with the mother: "From the depths of the sea surges a monster who terrifies us. It combines the maleficence of the subterranean world of the dead with the abjection of maternal ambivalences—persecuting power *and* castration" (2012, 29–30). Beyond this Freudian double valence, Kristeva wonders whether Medusa could be a symbol of humanity's attempt to separate from the animal and the individual subject's attempt to separate from the mother. In this way, Medusa becomes a representative, if not a representation, of both the cut or separation that is the primary trauma of the human condition, on the one hand, and its antidote, on the other. In other words, the decapitated Medusa is a figure for castration and cutting, and yet she has the power to castrate or cut. Furthermore, the association between Medusa and reflection, and the protection she offers through her image, shields us from the very trauma she "represents." Kristeva says, "a dialectic of representation is formed between Perseus and the Gorgon that reproduces the ambivalent passions of the mother-child separation. Fortunately, the give-and-take comes down to one brutal, simple solution: Medusa's gaze kills, but it is the *reflection*—the figure of splitting in two, of representation—that finally kills Medusa" (30).

Relying on Kristeva's theories of maternal abjection and separation in other works such as *Powers of Horror*, we can extend her analysis of Medusa as a figure of both separation from the maternal body and protection from that body through representation. It is through representing the maternal body that the child can come to love the mother. In other words, the child weans itself from the maternal body through an imaginary matricide, decapitation even, that prefigures the operations of language and representation themselves. Cutting and separation are necessary if the child is to become independent of the mother. Yet separation is also inherent in the operation of representation. The word or symbol stands in for what is absent or cut off, the thing. And for Kristeva that thing always takes us back to the first thing, the maternal body.

In her analysis of Freud's case of Little Hans, Kristeva argues that the child's first attempts to represent the world are telescoped substitutions for experiences that cannot be named, the unnamable, represented by what she calls the maternal hieroglyph. Ultimately, bodily experiences and sensations cannot be captured by words or representation; therefore our attempts to do so are always outstripped by those experiences. This is simultaneously why we continue to try and why we are doomed to fail. This is the cut, the separation, definitive of the human condition—and perhaps all life—that can be soothed, if only temporarily, through art and representation. The separation that is life, including the ultimate separation, death, becomes bearable only through representation. In Athena's rearview mirror we can face the horror, not head-on or frontally, but through its reflection and representations. Thus Kristeva suggests that images may "be the way to salvation" (2012, 31). Even if we cannot accept this redemptive view of images or art, they do have the power to make life—and death—more bearable. Even if they cannot save us from the pain and suffering of the cut, they allow us the possibility of reinterpretation over and over again, so that we can continue to suffer and continue to try to overcome that suffering through representing it.

Kristeva says, "Cut off Medusa's head and make it into a reflection if you want to see (it), if you want to know. Spectacle, speculation—whether erotic or philosophic—is rooted in your first triumphs over your archaic terrors. . . . Could Medusa be the patron goddess of visionaries and artists?" (2012, 33). Medusa as a figure for the maternal body, the maternal sex; Medusa as goddess; and Medusa as girl, as sister. Kristeva plays with the associations between Medusa and coral, which turns to stone when it is exposed to air; she points out that the Greek word *gorgonion* means coral, and she muses, "the generic word *coral* could come from *coré*, which means 'young girl'" (29). We are back to those mothers and girls who both threaten and erect both man's creativity and his sovereignty. Indeed, if we follow Kristeva, who associates Medusa with what she calls her "brutally erotic cousin" the praying mantis who devours her mate after sex, we have returned to the territory of the she-wolf, whose devouring mouth and fecund sex are threatening, yet (because they are) powerful. She also associates Medusa with Baubô, "castration compensated for by phallic simulacrum? Or, on the contrary, the phallic simulacrum revealing the abject power, not yet apparent, of the Mother possessor of life for death, prior to any capacity for representation?" (32). Kristeva points to this double aspect of Medusa as both life-bearing and death-bearing when she says, "vulva and vultus, genitals or face, two fantastical equivalents that the myth of Medusa brings together again thousands of years later. Vuvlar, phallic, necessitating, if not the erasure of the face, at least its decapitation so that a representation can take over, Medusa is essentially the iconic human experience" (32).

If art is like a Medusa that freezes and kills life, it is also life-giving, life-bearing. Like the scissors that cut for the sake of rebirth with and beyond death, the Medusa effect does both. Kristeva goes further: "mirror work and coral work. A secret genealogy between the power of Gorgons and the aesthetic experience follows the course of the centuries. It makes us understand that if artists manage to avoid being Medusa's victims, it is because they reflect her, even while being transubstantiations of her blood. The Medusa myth already prefigures an aesthetic of incarnation" (2012, 36). Leaving aside the religious intonation of her remarks, Kristeva wagers that art can lead to transformation and transubstantiation as rebirth with and through the cut, with and through death. Like Derrida, she is willing to take the gamble that aesthetic experience might allow us to glimpse what is beyond the machines of both nature and culture. The Medusa effect of art and poetic majesty may be powerful enough to take on death-bearing violence, whether it is given in so-called nature or made by man's so-called sovereignty.

PART THREE

Death Machines

FIVE

Elephant Autopsy: Optic Machinery and the Scale of Sovereignty

> One thinks of this elephenomenelephant that was no longer looking at them but could have seen them, with its own eyes seen the king see it in its own autopsy.
>
> —JACQUES DERRIDA, *The Beast and the Sovereign*

Derrida asks us to read (hear) his seminar *The Beast and the Sovereign* as a fable, similar to the fables of La Fontaine that punctuates the text. Just as La Fontaine's fables often employ two (or more) characters—animals—to teach us lessons about political power, the seminar is the story of two characters—two animals—the beast and the sovereign, engaged in a life-and-death struggle, in which the sovereign turns out to be the more beastly of the two. If Derrida's *Beast* is a fable, we might ask, what is its moral? What lessons are we to learn from it? In a word, we could say it is a lesson about the workings of sovereignty, but of course it is also much more. Indeed, it is a sort of counterfable set as counterweight to the fable of sovereignty, particularly the fable of human sovereignty over animals. Although various animals show up in this text (and in Derrida's work more generally), one story that illustrates some of the stakes of his counterfable about sovereignty is that of a big elephant and a little king. Derrida asks us to imagine the doctors, "or other armed butchers," "trembling with lust for autopsy," impatient to sink their axes and knifes into "the great defenseless body," while the diminutive king, Louis le Grand (Louis XIV), makes a grand entrance in great pomp and ceremony to inspect the "enormous, heavy, poor beast," an elephant who lived in the Versailles menagerie until "he" died in 1681 (2009, 284). Unlike the morals of La Fontaine's fables, however, the moral of this story is not obvious. Indeed, the circulation of the gaze required to prop up His Majesty the little king on the back, so to speak, of this great animal, this "elephenomenelephant," is head-spinning.

Like La Fontaine's fable "The Wolf and the Lamb" with which Derrida begins the seminar, and "The Heifer, the Goat, and the Ewe in Society with the Lion" that shows up later, this too is a story of *might makes right*. But unlike in those stories, in which the wolf and the lion are clearly the stronger of the animals (the lion threatens to devour the others, and the wolf makes good on the threat), here the giant elephant, which could crush the little king with one footfall, is lying at the foot of the strutting sovereign. There is no conversation, no debate, no outwitting or intimidating, as with La Fontaine's animals. Rather, there is a dead elephant at center stage, surrounded by the king and his court performing sovereignty in the autopsy chamber. Perhaps Derrida seeks to provide the kind of fabulous conversation that might lead to this scene of a mighty beast fallen before a puny man, the backstory of why and how this dead giant is needed in both the fable of the king's sovereignty over his subjects and the fable of man's sovereignty over other animals.

Although he claims that he too is engaging in fables, Derrida also insists on exposing the fable of sovereign political power *as fable* (exposure is a complicated gesture in the Derridean corpus), while trying to avoid fables that involve the fabulization of animals in "an anthropomorphic taming, a moralizing subjection, a domestication," which is part and parcel of the discourse of man's sovereignty over them (2008, 37). As a start, then, we could say that the moral of Derrida's counterfable of the elephant autopsy is that man's sovereignty comes at the price of animal lives; that man lives through killing animals. Moreover, the *political animal* in particular requires necropsy in order to sustain its political power. Furthermore, we could say that a certain sovereignty as necropsy erects itself through this autopsic model of power: "[W]e are dealing with a political organization of the field of knowledge, in the form of the anatomy lesson or the lesson of the natural sciences," that is, the autopsy (2009, 273). Like the fabled elephant who never forgets, Derrida does not let us forget that sovereign power is erected on death, particularly the death of animals, both the animals with whom we share the planet and the animals within us.

In this chapter, I take up what Derrida calls "the globalization of the autopsic model" of sovereignty in relation to the counterfable of the elephant autopsy (2009, 296). I consider the mechanism of the "sovereignty effect" of both king and man, and the sovereign power of both to lord over others, that requires a unique witness, and witnesses to that witness, in a circulation of the gaze that ends in autopsy. Sovereignty requires the spectacle or performance of sovereignty and the testimony of an intermediary both uniquely present at this performance and yet necessarily absent from the "official aesthetic" of sovereign rhetoric. Yet, as we will see, there is a blind spot in this sovereign gaze that again is both necessary and unsettling to it, namely, the dead eyes of that elephant lying in the theater of autopsy. The eyes of this "elephenomenelephant," with their ex-orbitant orbs in excess of what is proper to the limits of man, necessarily exceed the boundaries of the autopsic model of sovereignty; and, like the return of the repressed body, the body become corpse, they look back at the living even in death, not by yielding their secrets to the light, but rather by refusing the light with their opaqueness, these dead elephantine eyes. The secrets of this elephant, the secrets of life itself, do not yield to the autopsic gaze. Rather, there is always something beyond the limits of human seeing, something exorbitant, beyond the limits of human understanding, beyond human control, and beyond human mastery.

The Theater and Spectacle of Autopsy

Even as we define ourselves as human against both the animal and the machine, we cannot know for certain *who* we are or *what* they are; or that we can tell a *who* from a *what*. As we have seen, Derrida is not taking the all-too-simple line that we are animals or that we are machines, or that animals or robots are people too. He rejects that view as asinine. Rather, he is challenging the limits, the borders, and the border police, who insist on fixed categorical oppositions between *us* and *them* in order to justify building fences and walls, and worse, to justify building zoos, slaughterhouses, asylums, prisons, gas-chambers, and other beastly technologies of death. There is always something exorbitant, something that exceeds the limits and borders that we erect, most particularly the border between *us* and *them*.

The elephant autopsy points to one of the ways in which we justify our beastly treatment of *them*. In the name of knowledge and science we perform our lust for autopsy. Derrida's invocation of the elephant, however, also operates as a kind of eulogy to the exorbitant grandeur of the elephant that escapes the elephantine spectacle surrounding it through which the diminutive king asserts his power. Derrida asks us to imagine the scene and to remember this grand nameless beast, to see the scene from his (or her?) perspective. He follows the trace of the life's breath of this real big elephant, the invisible revenant beyond autopsy, the secrets of its life and death that remain unseen, beyond the scope or scale of humanity and its assertions of self-sovereignty. In a way, he asks us to mourn this grandest of animals, an animal also known for its capacity to mourn. Following Derrida, I suggest that mourning, particularly elephant mourning, is what resists autopsy, or at least it is what never fully yields to, or avails itself of, autopsy; there is always an other elephant, the real big elephant, the elephant revenant, that denies the satisfaction of autopsy and refuses to give up its secrets, whether it is the secret of what it is to be an elephant, or the secret of what it is to be an animal, or the secret of what it is to be a living being. Like the really real girl, or the real little cat, this is the elephant that looks back from its dead eyes to haunt the fable of the living sovereign. This is the counterfable of how an elephant eye puts out the "I" of sovereignty; it is another story of an *eye* for an *I*; another story of how one nail takes out another, which gives a new twist to *lex talionis*, or justice as retribution in the biblical "eye for an eye."

With the fable of the elephant and the king, Derrida shows how the quest for knowledge is driven by lust for autopsy, the desire to dissect the mysteries of life (and death) under a laboratory spotlight. It is a violent operation of subjecting everything to the tools of dissection, under glaring lights focused beneath the gaze of one who establishes himself as sovereign precisely through this gaze and the supposed mastery or knowledge it produces and that he supposedly possesses through it, exposing everything to "the violence of light" (cf. "Violence and Metaphysics" in Derrida 1978). The autopsic model of knowing is one of prying things open, exposing them to tools, light, and the scientific gaze, in order to determine the cause-and-effect relationships that supposedly explain our own existence. Today, autopsies are *performed* (note this turn of phrase) in cases, especially criminal and medical cases, in which the causes of death are unknown or uncertain. Forensic autopsies in particular are performed in order to solve the mystery of "who dunnit" and how. Autopsies are never performed for the sake of the dead, who can no longer benefit from them, but always for the sake of the living, for the sake of revenge, or justice as revenge, or for scientific knowledge that might benefit the living.

This couldn't be more obvious than in the case of the elephant autopsy, performed not for that nameless beast or even for his or her kind, but rather presumably to learn something about the functioning of the human body, and more especially, to entertain the king. More importantly, Derrida argues that the elephant autopsy performs the king's sovereignty over man and beast. The royal scientists and doctors are there at his behest, the spectators too, bowing before him, and the elephant is the carnage, literally, of this spectacle of sovereignty. Laid out in the theater of autopsy, the giant animal is a testament to the power of the king over the entire world, even the world of nature. Derrida contends that this scene is an emblem of the intimate connection between theory and theater, between speculation and spectacle: "[T]his optical, autoptical scene . . . makes use of an absolute power over the beast with a view to seeing and knowledge, in the name, at bottom, of Enlightenment, but of light, always that of the Sun King, light that in the end never dissociates theoretical observation in the service of knowledge, here for example the optics of autopsy—[never dissociates it] from spectacle, theater, ceremony as representation, and representation as representation *of* the king (a double genitive again), both the spectacular representation given by the king, ordered by him, organized by him in view of himself, and the representation *of* the king that represents the king, that presents him, shows him in his portrait, or recounts him in action" (2009, 287).

The etymological connection between *theory* and *theater* is played out in the scene of autopsy. First, as Derrida reminds us, the word *autopsy* is from the Latin *autopsia*, from *autos* (self) and *optos* (seen), to see with one's own eyes,[1] while the word *theory* is from the Greek *theoria*, which means contemplation or speculation, from *theoros*, which means spectator, to see with the mind's eye. And *speculation* and *spectacle* both have the same Latin root, *specere*, which means to look. Indeed, *speculation* comes from *specula*, the word for watchtower as a vantage point high above from which to look down and see not only the lay of the land, but also approaching enemies—speculation as a means of defense. Both theoretical observation and philosophical speculation, then, have their roots in *looking*, observing from on high, from the vantage point of the king, or at least of the king's watchman. Theory, speculation, and autopsy are modes of seeing, either as eyewitness or with the mind's eye. The spectacle of death, now transferred to the theater of autopsy, plays out the morbid curiosities of all those present to it, all those interested in seeing; and who can resist? Judging by the popularity of spectacles of death and autopsy scenes in popular television and film, no one can resist. Yet, as we will see (so to speak), the exorbitant eyes of the dead elephant have a look beyond the limits of our vision, of our looking, of our autopsic gaze.

Following his friend and colleague Louis Marin's *Portrait of the King*, Derrida traces the circulation of the autopsic gaze in this unholy scene that ordains the king as Lord of the Land. Marin argues that although the king's history must be narrated from the God's-eye-view in order to transfer the power of absolute sovereignty from that point of view onto the king, the narrator who speaks from that position must disappear from the narrative.[2] In other words, the historian himself must not be seen to be seeing the king. He must exhibit what Derrida calls the *visor effect* wherein he sees without being seen, as if he is wearing a suit of armor through which he sees but cannot be seen.[3]

Re-presentation and re-production operate through revealing and concealing the death of the very thing they supposedly present as living. This is the paradox of representation and of testimony. As Marin's analysis makes clear, this paradox of representation is further complicated in the case of the king, insofar as the king's portrait not only anticipates the king's death, such that all representations of the king are of a dead rather than living king, but also his historian and portrait painter must die too in the act of turning the first-person account into a third-person one. In other words, there can be no "I" in the king's performance of sovereignty. Or, more precisely, his "I" must be reported by a third party who hides himself; and it is this third party who is truly the bearer of the visor effect that produces the illusion of the king's sovereignty. He is the bearer of the gaze that must not be *seen seeing* and yet must testify to his privileged seeing.

Derrida attributes the visor effect to the king (in *Specters of Marx*, to the ghostly king returning to haunt Hamlet) as evidence of the asymmetry of the gaze required to maintain sovereignty. This optics of *hyperoptics*, as he calls it, marks the sovereign "by the power to see, by being-able-to-see without being seen. . . . [T]he king or the king's specter sees without his gaze, the origin of his seeing, without his eyes being seen" (2009, 293). Certainly this is true of the king's gaze at the dead elephant. In an absolute sense, the elephant cannot see the king looking at it; and moreover, the king's gaze upon the mammoth creature establishes his power over it. There is an absolute asymmetry of the gaze.

Yet for Marin, the king's visibility is also essential to his power, which is not quite the visor effect. The king is visible, but always and only through an intermediary. His subjects must not look directly at him. He alone has the sovereign power to look directly at them. He is the bearer of the gaze and they are its objects. So, while the king does hide behind an armor, so to speak, he not only sees without being seen, but also must be seen seeing for the effects of his image to work their magic and produce the very sovereignty they seem to re-present. This is not lost on Derrida, who, like Marin, attempts to shine the light on sovereignty itself—or, as Derrida says, perform an autopsy on autopsy—and bring into the light the interludes in the *performance* of sovereignty as narrative fiction; there would be no sovereignty without the representation of it (2009, 289). It is fabular, a fabulous fable.

Derrida extends Marin's analysis of the transfer of sovereign power from the monarchy to democracy through the circulation of proclamations of sovereignty. He claims that although the Sun King Louis XIV's grandson, Louis XVI, was subjected to the guillotine that began the bloody Reign of Terror of the French Revolution, which eventually produced the Rights of Man and government by the people, the mechanics of sovereignty did not change. Today's representatives of the people, presidents, prime ministers, and politicians, are just as caught up in erecting their sovereignty through the image as was King Louis XIV and his extraordinary elephant; or his son, Louis XV, the Monseigneur le Dauphin to whom La Fontaine dedicated his political fables, already using the panegyric rhetoric memorializing the future king's eternal body by imagining the death of his earthly one: "I invoke as testimony those noble worries, that vivacity, that ardor, those marks of spirit, of courage and of grandeur of soul [the kid is six and a half] that you show at every moment" (quoted in Derrida 2009, 212; bracketed comment is Derrida's). With televisual media, politicians are more conscious than ever about the need to control "their constituents" by controlling the media and the circulation of images. Democracy has not changed this certain sovereignty, whereby the performance of might makes right and the official aesthetic makes and breaks "kings."

In his deconstruction of this certain sovereignty, Derrida exposes sovereignty as the performance of sovereignty, as in La Fontaine's fable "The Heifer, the Goat, and the Ewe in Society with the Lion," in which the lion asserts or performs his sovereignty by proclaiming it: "I am Lion." In other words, sovereignty is a linguistic performance, like the pronouncement *I do* in the marriage ceremony; the saying *I am sovereign* is the doing of it, the making it so. Yet Marin emphasizes another element essential to this performative declaration, namely, that it must have an audience or a witness. In the case of the lion, it is the three girls, the heifer, the goat, and the ewe, who are witnesses to his declarations of sovereignty, and their presence is part of the circulation of the gaze that props up sovereignty.

Sovereignty, then, is not only a performance in the linguistic sense of saying as doing, but also in the theatrical sense of putting on a show for an audience. The sovereign is nothing without his subjects; his glory must be witnessed. This creates the paradox of sovereignty: the king must be seen seeing and yet not be seen (for what he really is, a mortal man, especially a mortal animal among others). His subjects must not look at him directly, which is why he can be seen only through an intermediary, a representation, a portrait, narrative or otherwise. Even the ceremonial scene of the elephant autopsy is staged so that the king can be seen seeing and the deadly power of his seeing can be witnessed. This is why the role of the historian or the portrait artist is essential to the operations of sovereignty. (Today photography, television, and the internet supplement the historian and portraiture.) The king needs an intermediary to represent his sovereignty, to witness him proclaiming it, to witness to it "directly." This witness, however, must efface himself in the process, so that his portrait is seen as if it were the king himself. In this way, the king's person, his body, is also disregarded for the sake of his eternal royal body as both sovereign monarch and sacred representative of God on earth.[4]

The paradoxical effect is that the king's greatness, his majesty, must be witnessed "directly" through the representations of it by eyewitnesses who adopt the position of God or history itself in order to create the sovereign-effect in the viewer/listener. The mediation is required to create the effect of immediacy. This is the paradox of witnessing that Derrida discusses in his work on testimony. The eyewitness always testifies to something that he saw with his own eyes but is now absent. His report is taken as evidence of the immediacy of a past that he experienced in a unique way that is both singular and yet repeatable in the testimony. In other words, the testimony and the act of testifying assume that the witness can relay events or repeat them, at the same time that they assume that the events are not repeatable insofar as he is unique in his capacity as witness. Derrida forcefully describes this paradox in *The Instant of My Death/Demeure*: "When I testify, I am unique and irreplaceable. And at the very tip of this irreplaceability, this unicity, once again, there is the instant. Even if we have been several to participate in an event, to have been present at a scene, the witness can only testify when he asserts that he was in a unique place and where he could testify to this and that in a here-now, that is, in a pointed instant that precisely supports this exemplarity. The example is not substitutable; but at the same time the same aporia always remains: this irreplaceability must be exemplary, that is, replaceable. The irreplaceable must allow itself to be replaced on the spot. . . . The singular must be universalizable; this is the testimonial condition" (2000, 41). The condition of the possibility of testimony—its uniqueness and irreplaceability—is destroyed by the act of testimony itself (cf. 2000, 33).

This paradox at the heart of witness is the problem of technology that Derrida discusses throughout his work and that we have been analyzing throughout this book. In what we take to be natural, there is already a technological supplement. In what we take to be original, there is already a copy. Indeed, the copy or reproduction produces the effect of originality and nature. So too with the eyewitness. What the witness sees with his own eyes must be reported, and in that testimony it must be put into words or images that reproduce it through so many technologies, even more so today when technologies of reproduction are multiplying. Derrida says, "The technical reproducibility is excluded from testimony, which always calls for the presence of the live voice in the first person. But from the moment that a testimony must be able to be repeated, techne is admitted; it is introduced where it is excluded" (2000, 42; cf. 2002a, 98). Reproduction is always mediated by technology, by the machine, and is never the result of something purely natural in itself, whether we are talking about the reproduction of texts and images or the reproduction of plants and animals, as we have seen, most especially of human animals. What we take to be natural is an effect of this witnessing process that involves re-presentation and re-production as the circulation of sovereignty, of the "I can" in "I can see for myself" or "I can tell the truth." And it is always a performative gesture based on faith rather than on *cold hard facts* as evidence (cf. Derrida 2002a). Indeed, the witness always risks becoming a mere answering machine, repeating the same story over and over again until it becomes the Truth (cf. 2002a, 100).

Recall that for Freud, the introduction of re-production and re-presentation moves humanity from mere animals into civilization and becomes the grounds for patriarchy. For him, the male organ represents the ultimate witness as a symbol of fertility, while the female remains like an animal in her relation to childbirth. In *Totem and Taboo*, he describes the movement to human civil society in terms of the fraternal horde overpowering the primal father and substituting the animal totem for him. For Freud, civilization begins with this violent substitution through which the dead father becomes more powerful that the living one ever was. The absent father and his imagined virility are the grounds for the patriarchal law that follows. The etymological connection between *testimony*, which comes from the Latin root *testis*, confirms the privilege of the phallus in representation as reproduction. The very word for witness contains the male organ, *testis*, as witness to virility. And, on Freud's account, the power and virility of the primal father is realized only through the totemic representations of him and the ritualized repetitions of the primal murder. Here again, the sovereign's inaugural power comes from the representation and assimilation of his dead body (not to mention the dead bodies of animals).

Marin's theory of the king's three bodies explains how sovereign power belongs to the dead rather than the living king or sovereign; or, we could say, the king or sovereign's power necessarily assumes his death. Revising Ernst Kantorowicz's theory of the two bodies of the king, his natural body and his political body, to incorporate the power of the image, Marin identifies three bodies: the mortal (animal) body, the juridical political body, and the sacramental body represented in images, both narrative and visual. The operation of the juridical political body depends upon the "death" of the mortal animal body, or at least its transformation into the sacramental body depicted in the history and portraits of the king. This third body guarantees the king's sovereign power by replacing, or standing in for, the other two bodies, or what Marin says unifies the three. It is this third body, the image of the king, which makes him eternal. Through these images, the king becomes what he is as a benevolent or feared ruler overlooking his subjects from on high, particularly as he looks out from his portrait over the heads of his subjects. His unseeing eyes survey his entire kingdom and ensure that he can be everywhere at once, that he is erected as sovereign across his kingdom.

Derrida links the three bodies of the king to three meanings of the word *autopsy*, a word that, he points out, Marin also uses to describe princely power as enacted through a sort of eulogy before death.[5] This eulogy is the narrative produced by the "invisible" historian—flattery posing as fact, which in effect "kills" the king's earthly, mortal animal body and replaces it with an eternal sovereign body, which in turn authorizes his juridical political body. This form of "ancient autopsy" is the demand that the narrative of past events be authenticated by an eyewitness, in this case the king's narrator, who serves as "a 'witness' or even a 'martyr' (originally the same thing)" (Derrida 2009, 294). In the sense that the narrator must make himself absent for the sake of making the king's presence absolute through his narrative, he does martyr himself. This sense of the word *autopsy* is a literal sense of seeing with one's own eyes. But Derrida points out that there are two other meanings, one rare and one current. *Autopsy* also means participation in the omnipotence of the gods, which is what authorizes all narratives of absolute sovereignty. And it has come to mean the dissection of a cadaver, or necropsy.

All three of these meanings converge on the sovereignty of the king produced through his three bodies and symbolized by the elephant autopsy, with its big animal and little king. The mortal body is there in the dead elephant: "This dead elephant . . . the denied averted, vaguely totemic representation of the dead king, the mortal king, the king dead from a death . . . that every subject projects into the autopsy or the necropsy of sovereignty" (2009, 294). Since the word *elephant* can refer not only to the pachyderm but also to a big man, in the sense of someone important, the elephant is not just any animal double.[6] The spectacle of autopsy itself authorizes the king's juridical or sovereign body. And the king's eternal body is created through the representation of the spectacle. The resplendent story of the scene of the autopsy with its great pomp and ceremony creates the autopsy as participation in the eternal power of a god. And, that, in turn, authorizes the witness to tell the story as the truth of His Majesty's greatness and thereby produce the sovereign effect through the representation itself. The omnipotence of gods is reflected and deflected through the narrative that both divides and produces its power. The sovereignty effect is the effect of death, both in the real body of the once-majestic animal lying on the operating table in pieces, and in the symbolic body that replaces the mortal body of the king. The king's mortality, then, is doubly displaced in this scene of autopsy—perhaps infinitely divisible and displaced in the circulation of representation that produces sovereignty and the sovereign-effect.[7]

The three bodies and three autopsies they entail are at the heart of the opposition between the beast and the sovereign, between animal and man. For, if within the official aesthetic, the king has three bodies (sacred, soul, and mortal body), we could say that the ordinary man has two (soul and mortal body), while animals have only one (mortal body). Indeed, the mortal body of the king, his earthly finite body, is his animal body; and this body is always the animal that must be sacrificed for society and humanity. Recall that in the story of Freud's primal horde, it is the animal body that is sacrificed for the sake of the body memorialized through symbols, particularly the totem; and this is how *homo sapiens* became civilized social humans. The mortal body has been associated with the animal, and it has been sacrificed to gods, to science, and to culture. Within the fable of human sovereignty, the sacrifice of the elephant in the spectacle of the elephant autopsy is a necessary part of the process of turning the animal *homo sapiens* into a man and turning a man into a king. In the case of the king, it also requires the third body, the one witnessed and thereby authorized by eternity through the portrait that turns the performance of sovereignty into history. It all begins with the metaphorical death of his animal body—and the literal death of other animal bodies, which are seen as merely bodies and nothing more—for the sake of his eternal soul.

"Just to See . . ."

Indeed, these animals bodies killed so that we might become human are not only sacrificed to God in our stead (Freud's totemic animal and the stories of Genesis), or used by us for food and clothing, but are also subjected to scientific research in laboratories. The scientific study of animals, which has a history dating back at least to ancient Greece, not only provides us with shampoos that don't irritate our eyes and give us silkier hair, but also feeds our hunger for knowledge. The lust for autopsy as the lust for knowledge is supposedly one characteristic that separates us from other animals. We are burning with longing to know, to understand, to unlock the secrets of life. Other animals are presumed to be content to live it rather than understand it or imagine it otherwise. We, on the other hand, require another life beyond our animal mortality to make it worthwhile. This is the driving force behind both science and religion, namely, the demand for an explanation beyond this life itself, a life beyond life. For science this means dissecting everything, exposing it to the "violence of light" just in order to satisfy our curiosity about how the universe works—"just to see," as Derrida repeatedly says in *The Animal that Therefore I Am*. For religion this means belief in a transcendent God greater than us, an absolute sovereign, whose mysteries we cannot know but must accept on faith. In either case, we look for a life beyond life, beyond our mere mortal animal bodies. Both take their revenge, so to speak, on the body, particularly the body in pieces or cut up. Scientists dissect the body to examine every bit of it; nothing is sacred. Whereas religious violence continues to target the integrity of the body through spectacles of beheadings, rapes, and tortures (see 2002a, 88). More and more there is a paradoxical convergence of holy wars and techno-science, which make religion another scopic machine of death (see 2002a, 82).

In "Faith and Knowledge," Derrida maintains that there is a double mechanics at work here, a machine that reproduces death for the sake of life: "I refer to it as mechanics because it reproduces, with the regularity of a technique, the instance of the non-living or, if you prefer, of the dead in the living" (2002a, 86). It is the deadly machine of life. This mechanism of reproducing death at the heart of life is the motor of the killing machine of both science and religion insofar as both require the death of the earthly body: science in the name of autopsy, dissection, and knowledge, and religion in the name of heaven, an afterlife, and God.

This death at the heart of life has been the subject of Derrida's deconstructive project since its beginnings. More recently, he turned the deconstruction machine against this killing machine as it manifests itself in discourses (or fables and fictions) through which killing is justified as right, whether in science, religion, or law. For example, in "Faith and Knowledge," he dismantles the machine as it operates in religion and in philosophy as the double movement of sanctity of life on the one hand, and righteous killing on the other. In the essay, he sees in the fundamentalist prohibitions against abortion, artificial insemination, gene therapies, and stem cell research the extension of the universal commandment "Thou shalt not kill," which seems at odds with the equally universal commandment "An eye for an eye," or *lex talionis*, which demands the death penalty in the name of God, not to mention other biblical proclamations that give man dominion over all the animals of the earth to dispose of as he will, including in slaughterhouses and factory farms (see Derrida 2002a, 86). Although these religious principles seem at odds with each other, many Christian fundamentalists comfortably protest against abortion while advocating for the death penalty. Derrida's explanation for this tension is the "auto-immunity" of religion, working against its own most universal principles in a mechanics that turns religious fundamentalists and fanatics into machines, deadly machines acting out these conflicting principles as if programmed to do so by the ultimate computer programmer, God himself.[8]

There is a hatred of life diagnosed by Nietzsche at work here that places the value of life beyond life, in both celebrating the death of the (animal) body and imagining ourselves always already dead and gone to heaven. Derrida identifies this mechanism with an infinite mourning, which is, we might say, both mourning for the life that is killed off for the sake of another, the life of the body, and mourning for the life we long for that is not yet ours, not until we kill off the animal within us—mourning for eternal life or absolute knowledge.[9] Derrida puts it differently: "the marionette, the dead machine yet more than living, the spectral fantasy of the dead as the principle of life and of sur-vival [*sur vie*]. This mechanical principle is apparently very simple: life has absolute value only if it is worth *more than* life. And hence only in so far as it mourns, becoming itself in the labour of infinite mourning, in the indemnification of a spectrality without limit" (2002a, 87). Putting the value of life beyond life leads to an eternal ideal world beyond this one, which in turn leads to an infinite mourning for the absolute discrepancy between this world and the next, between the real world and the ideal one. In this way, in this perverse view, only through death (the death of the real in favor of the ideal) does life become worthy of its name, Life.

As we have seen, sovereignty and the circulation of the gaze that supports it requires the death of the mortal animal body and the fantasy of a dead king who becomes more powerful through this imagined death than he is as a living person. The "spectrality without limit" resonates with Marin's analysis of the power of the image of the dead—or always-already-dead—king. It also recalls the power of Freud's absent totemic father to be greater than the real father, to be more powerful as a symbol than he was as a living animal. In both cases, mourning is what intensifies the power of the image or representation that both makes die and makes live forever. The performance of sovereignty, which necessitates this infinite mourning of the always-already-dead sovereign through his third body or sacred image, shares with the religious desire for another life and with the scientific desire for absolute knowledge a lust for autopsy that requires the death and dissection of the earthly animal body for the sake of human sovereignty, whether that sovereignty is evidenced by man's dominion over other animals, his immortal soul, or his capacity for knowledge. Indeed, religion and science both rely on the sacrifice of animal bodies for the sake of propping up human exceptionalism and our right to use animals. Traditionally, our dominion over them has been so absolute that killing animals was not seen as true killing, and certainly not as murder or warfare, because animals as bodies are always already merely corpses anyway; or as Descartes imagines them, mere soulless machines. We might ask, however: Can animals have corpses? Or are they rather mere carcasses, the term *corpse* being reserved for humans? Heidegger, for example, maintains that animals do not die, but rather merely perish, because they have no knowledge of death, no being-toward-death, which is the special privilege or burden of Dasein. He also privileges man's hands, equipped with opposable thumbs, as both literal and metaphorical tools for grasping what other animals cannot. Dasein is out of their reach. And, as such (which for Heidegger is precisely what is at stake—the "as such," and animals' inability to grasp life or death "as such"), for Heidegger, animals have no relation to death and therefore no possibility of mourning. They are absolutely excluded from the possibility of the infinite mourning necessary for the performance of sovereignty, and thereby excluded from any possibility of representation or culture.

Elephantine Mourning

Derrida challenges the traditional belief, shared by Heidegger, that only humans die, that only *we* are capable of mourning, and that only *we* perform rituals of mourning and bury our dead (see Derrida 2011, 41). Reading Heidegger in one hand and *Robinson Crusoe* in the other (as he says in *The Beast and the Sovereign*, vol. 2), Derrida quotes Leopold Bloom of James Joyce's *Ulysses*: "Only man buries. No ants do. First thing strikes anybody"; and then Derrida comments, "an error by Joyce who thinks like everyone else that beasts do not die in the proper sense, do not wear mourning and do not bury" (2010, 41; 2011, 17). Derrida is clear that he thinks it is an error to deny animals death properly speaking, mourning, or burial. When it comes to animals, Derrida's deconstructive strategy is to question both whether humans are properly capable of being-toward-death *as such* (in Heidegger's sense), mourning, or burying, and whether animals are not capable of death, mourning, or burying, *as such*. He refuses the absolute limit between human death, mourning, and burial and animal perishing without mourning or rituals around death. This is not to say that animals are people too, but rather, as Derrida repeatedly reminds us, to multiply the limits and borders between the overly general category *animal* and the overly exclusive category *man*. Derrida leaves open the possibility that animals know death, mourn their dead, and engage in burial rituals.

Was the fabled elephant laid out on the autopsy table before Louis le Grand mourned by his family and friends? Did they protest against the lack of a proper burial for their kin—as a group of zoo elephants supposedly did until the bones of their dead companion were brought back into their enclosure so they could properly mourn?[10] Did his (or her) elephant friends give eulogies for him (or her), their now forever-absent colleague? After all, elephants too are known to mourn their dead with elaborate rituals that go on for years. One elephant researcher concludes, "Perhaps more than any other quality, the elephant is thought of as having understanding of death. Grieving and mourning rituals are an integral part of elephant culture" (Bradshaw 2004, 147). And discussing research on elephants, a reporter concludes, "When an elephant dies, its family members engage in intense mourning and burial rituals, conducting weeklong vigils over the body, carefully covering it with earth and brush, revisiting the bones for years afterward, caressing the bones with their trunks, often taking turns rubbing their trunks along the teeth of a skull's lower jaw, the way living elephants do in greeting" (Siebert 2006, 4). According to another elephant expert, elephants "have a memory that far surpasses ours and spans a lifetime [70 years]. They grieve deeply for lost loved ones, even shedding tears and suffering depression" (Sheldrick 1992). There is even a recent report of two herds of wild South African elephants traveling for twelve hours to visit the house of late author and elephant conservationist Lawrence Anthony upon his death. Anthony's family has no idea how the elephants, most of whom he saved and then returned to the wild, knew he had died. But within days of his death, two herds arrived within a day of each other, both in single file as if in a funeral procession, and stayed at the house, perhaps in vigil, for two days before returning to the bush.[11] This suggests that elephants may have more complicated capacities for mourning than humans have.

Elephants mourn their dead using their trunks, an appendage so utterly unfamiliar to us, so uncanny in its ability to grasp without those privileged opposable thumbs, without hands or arms. What is a trunk? And how would we measure up on the scale of the trunk? On the scale of the elephant, we are small enough to be crushed with one footfall. And even the grandest of human hands are unable to fully grasp the trunk, at least not without cutting it into pieces through dissection or ripping those magnificent ivory tusks from it.

Indeed, much recent research on elephants suggests that elephants possess many of the characteristics traditionally reserved for humans, including memory, self-awareness, emotions, attachment, social bonds, mourning, stress, trauma, communication, humor, and other complex behaviors and social structures.[12] Neuroscientists have established changes in elephants' brains after trauma, and they have discovered that elephants have an "extremely large and convoluted hippocampus that is responsible for mediating long-term social memory" (Bradshaw and Shore 2007, 432; cf. Siebert 2011). "Studies show that structures in the elephant brain are strikingly similar to those in humans. MRI scans of an elephant's brain suggest a large hippocampus, the component in the mammalian brain linked to memory and an important part of its limbic system, which is involved in processing emotions. The elephant brain has also been shown to possess an abundance of the specialized neurons known as spindle cells, which are thought to be associated with self-awareness, empathy and social awareness in humans. Elephants have even passed the mirror test of self-recognition, something only humans, and some great apes and dolphins, had been known to do" (Siebert 2011, 54). Some of these studies suggest that elephants have even better long-term memories, particularly social memories, than humans.

It has become a cliché that "elephants never forget," suggesting something like an animal archive, the perfect animal-memory machine, a mammoth memory, or the fable of the elephant. This fabulous elephant memory, bigger than life, is exorbitant insofar as we cannot comprehend another mammal with a lifelong memory, perhaps even better than our own. At the same time (or perhaps as a way of burying our own lack of understanding), the elephant becomes the fabular emblem of memory, the fabled animal against which Derrida works his counterfable, exemplified in his dissection of the fabled elephant autopsy.

This elephant subjected to the autopsic gaze of both science and sovereignty is cut apart for the sake of human knowledge and power. It performs an anatomy lesson in the theater of science as a body so large that it feeds not only our desire to see the size of its parts but also our desire for trophies of our triumph over the animal kingdom. Through this performance, as we have seen, man becomes the king of the beasts, while the diminutive Louis becomes the king of men. This fabled elephant becomes part of the symbolic exchange that produces sovereign power.

But what about the "real" elephant that died, or was killed, and somehow hauled into the autopsy chamber? Can we mourn the nameless elephant on the autopsy table even as "he" represents all elephants, all brains and muscles, and even Louis the Grand himself? According to Gustav Loisel, upon whose 1912 report Henri Ellenberger (1960) and then Derrida (2009) rely, the elephant lying on the autopsy table reportedly was a trickster with a sense of humor who lived thirteen years at the Versailles menagerie until "he" died in 1681; only at the autopsy did they discover that "he" was really a female elephant who apparently died of natural causes, or perhaps due to captivity (Loisel 1912, 115–18). How can we mourn that singular "real big elephant" lying before Louis XIV? Who can mourn this nameless elephant?[13] This question raises the larger question of whether or not we can mourn for animals. Certainly human grief over the loss of an animal companion can be as profound as the mourning for the loss of any other loved one. Yet mourning our animal loves is often seen as excessive or even unacceptable. There is little room for such mourning in the institutions of our culture. Perhaps, then, we are not as capable of mourning and grief as we think we are.

Did the fabled elephant—or any of the other elephants killed for ivory or for other human purposes—receive a proper burial? Elephants are known to bury even the dead of other species, particularly humans, especially when they kill them. They have been seen burying dead humans and performing mourning and burial rituals for them.[14] Do we do the same for them? Elephants have even been called in to resolve human-elephant conflict (HEC) as special Elephant Response Units (ERUs).[15] Human-elephant conflict is becoming more common as elephant habitat is taken over for human use, and poachers continue to ravage elephant populations, particularly targeting older elephants with bigger tusks. One elephant researcher describes a "war" against elephants, because humans "just throw hand grenades at the elephants, bring whole families down and cut out the ivory. I call that mass destruction" (see Siebert 2006). Various studies show that when the elders of a group of elephants are murdered, the young, especially the orphans, develop post-traumatic stress disorders and can become very aggressive against each other and other species, especially against other pachyderms and humans (Bradshaw 2004 and 2007; Siebert 2006 and 2011).[16] The *New York Times Magazine* article entitled "An Elephant Crack-Up?" that brought this phenomenon to public attention a few years ago opened with a close-up photograph of a long-lashed, welling, amber elephant eye, black pupil staring right into the camera, tears rolling down over the wrinkled, scaly pachyderm skin.

Did our fabled elephant shed tears facing its death? Did its elephant friends cry for it? Can we? Can we shed tears for this elephant or others, so different from us, without reducing them to fables that embody qualities we value in ourselves? Can we look at elephants with compassion instead of the lust for autopsy or the lust for ivory? What do we see when we look into the eye of an elephant? Or, more to the point, what does the elephant see when it looks at us? Can the gaze of an elephant, like the gaze of Derrida's cat in *The Animal that Therefore I Am*, "be, deep within her eyes, my primary mirror?" (2008, 51). This may be especially apt since it has been acknowledged that elephants share with humans the ability to recognize themselves in mirrors (Siebert 2011, 54). And what of the eyes of that poor beast, the dead elephant? What does that grandest of animals, that singular specimen, see through those dead eyes? Can those dead eyes be our mirrors? In passing, Derrida imagines an outrageous reversal of the gaze: "One thinks of this elephenomenelephant that was no longer looking at them but could have seen them, with its own eyes seen the king see it in its own autopsy" (2009, 282). What could this possibly mean—a dead elephant seeing the king looking, seeing the king usurping its grandeur through his autopsic gaze? What is the inversion of the gaze imagined by Derrida in this curious moment in *The Beast and the Sovereign*? We may get some clues from the "By Force of Mourning," a eulogy for his friend and colleague Louis Marin, particularly from Derrida's analysis there of the "inversion of the gaze" necessary for the "failure" of mourning, which is to say, any mourning worthy of its name.[17] This operation of inversion would also be the excess or remainder of mourning beyond all autopsy, what absolute sovereignty cannot allow, but is haunted by nonetheless.[18]

Mourning escapes autopsy insofar as the revenant returns in its singularity, its irreplaceability, this impossible repetition of what cannot be repeated, *this* elephant, this very one, like Derrida's "real little cat" who remains nameless in *The Animal that Therefore I Am* because to name is already to kill, to replace, to substitute. It is to substitute an eternal symbolic body for the mortal animal body, the body that is irreplaceable and therefore always also beyond the name, worthy of its name only insofar as it cannot be named. Its life and breath cannot be dissected. A "failed" mourning would be an elephant mourning, perhaps even a fabled or impossible mourning, one that does not and cannot forget; one that never ends. This "failed" mourning is not the melancholia that Freud opposes to remembering or working through, melancholia as a form of repetition. For what is mourned, the singular living being now forever gone, cannot be repeated. Only his image can be. Only in the ways in which he is appropriated by the machines of nature (genetics) and culture (books or creations) is he reproduced; never as the living, breathing, singular being he once was. It is to *this* revenant that Derrida appeals, to the other who resists assimilation or incorporation—not to the ghost, the specter or the phantom, those *visible* apparitions that appear to bring the dead back to life. What remains invisible, secret, unavailable to autopsy, is the life-breath of that now-dead elephant. The revenant haunts us with what cannot be seen, the irreplaceability of this elephant, that returns to us even now in Derrida's counterfable of the elephant and the king, but only as a trace.

"Successful" mourning, which is to say not mourning at all, is a type of autopsy insofar as it replays the absent other as so many memories, like pictures or movies shown on an interior screen. It subjects the other to the light of memory as a series of images, sometimes literally photographs or videos, intended to conjure the visage, the face of the beloved. But the revenant resists this autopsic model of mourning, of conjuring ghosts or apparitions, because it can only be felt and not seen—perhaps like the trunk of an elephant reaching for its dead friend or beloved. It cannot be projected onto the interior screen of *my* mind. Rather, it keeps its secrets and thereby takes me out of *my* mind, knocks *me* off *my* head, that capital representative of sovereignty and of philosophy.

Elephantine Revenant

Derrida argues that unlike the phantasm, specter, or ghost, the revenant does not appear; it does not make itself visible and therefore capable of capture or mastery by our senses; it cannot be brought into the light or placed under the autopsic gaze. Rather, the revenant "arises where there is no horizon. . . . [I]t allows itself to be dominated neither by a gaze, nor by a conscious perception in general, nor by a performative act of language. . . . The 'revenant,' however, comes and comes back (since singularity as such implies repetition) like the 'who' or 'what' of an event without a horizon. Like death itself" (2004, 230–31 fn. 34).[19] Specifically, Derrida describes the inversion of the gaze through which his dead friend Louis Marin looks at him as the gaze of the revenant. He says that the revenant looks at me, and not I at him; he interpolates me; I do not assimilate, introject, or incorporate him. Furthermore, the nonappearance of the revenant as event without horizon, as the secret that escapes autopsy, also shatters the interior space imagined to screen memories like so many picture-shows of the mind. The inversion of the gaze that comes to us from the other is not a reciprocal looking. Neither is it the circulation of the gaze of the sovereign that moves from the dead elephant, to the king, to the witnesses, to the court historian, to the reading/listening public (or to Loisel, to Ellenberger, through Marin, to Derrida, to us, etc.). It is not the gaze that establishes sovereignty—the "I can"—but precisely its inversion, what smashes the "I can" and "traumatizes the interiority that it inhabits" (Derrida 2001, 160). Death describes the alterity of the other as infinitely out of our reach, just as much in death as it was in life. Life (and death) keeps it secrets from the prying eyes of autopsy. It remains uncanny even in the scene of autopsy, perhaps especially in the scene of the elephant autopsy with its grand beast and diminutive sovereign. It puts out the *I* of the *I can* and takes us out of our mind, particularly insofar as we imagine ourselves in possession of a mind's eye. The gaze of the revenant puts out the mind's eye. This is a counterfable to the fable of an eye for an eye or *lex talionis*.

Reading the work of the late Marin, Derrida concludes, "However narcissistic it may be, our subjective speculation can no longer seize and appropriate this gaze before which we appear at the moment when, bearing it in us, bearing it along with every movement of our bearing or comportment, we can get over our mourning *of him* only by getting over *our* mourning, by getting over, by ourselves, the mourning of ourselves, I mean the mourning of our autonomy, of everything that would make us the measure of ourselves" (2001c, 160–61). How do we bear it? The excess of this absence, a hole in the heart, the exorbitant gaze of the revenant that unsettles rather than recalls us to ourselves as sovereign agents? Derrida maintains that this absence does not wait for death: "This 'mourning effect' thus does not wait for death. One does not wait for the death of the other to deaden and absorb his alterity. Faithfulness prescribes to me at once the necessity and the impossibility of mourning. It enjoins me to take the other within me, to make him live in me, to idealize him, to internalize him, but it also enjoins me not to succeed in the work of mourning: the other must remain the other" (2004, 160). This necessity but impossibility of assimilating the other makes mourning akin to eating, as analyzed in Derrida's "Eating Well." Since we must mourn the other, it is a question of how we do so. Do we mourn the other through autopsy as a defense against its life as it has lived it? Or do we engage in the infinite and interminable mourning for the secrets of its life that are lost to us forever, and always have been? In other words, do we respect its secrets and its otherness and welcome it even though we have not invited it, even though to do so endangers our own sense of ourselves as sovereign?

In sum, autopsy is just one way of avoiding the event of death, which is also to say the event of life, which is to say the event of mourning. The court scientists and the king look in vain at the remains of the grand beast without seeing the remainder always outside of their vision, the excess of life and death that resists their gaze and their sovereignty. They make a scene in order to cover up the fact that they cannot see what they are looking for, that the elephant refuses to reveal the secrets of his life, or more to the point, of life itself. The animal body refuses to yield all of its secrets to autopsy, whether that of the scientist as eyewitness or that of the philosopher gazing with his mind's eye.[20] Even the elephant's dead, blind eye sees more than they know, in Derrida's counterfantasy of the gaze of the revenant.

The gaze of the revenant shatters the hall of mirrors, the Cartesian theater of theory and speculation, in which the *cogito* thinks it reflects only itself without any other, its own sovereignty, that clearest and most distinct of ideas, *cogito ergo sum* (2004, 4).[21] The *cogito* is another scopic machine of death, the mind's eye, focused on itself, making of itself a dead object, not unlike the elephant carcass exposed to the glaring lights of autopsy. An *I* for an *eye*. That is the calculated exchange in the economy of sovereignty, the eye of an elephant for the I of a king. But not without remainder. Perhaps, then, the moral of Derrida's counterfable of the grand beast and the diminutive sovereign, the big elephant and the little king, is that like an elephant, we mustn't forget the remains of that "elephenomenelephant". . . the lost "real" elephant as a revenant that haunts our fable of sovereignty, and our fable of elephant memory and of elephant mourning, even as we struggle to use one fable to take out the other.

It is ironic that because elephants have very poor eyesight, they rely on touch, smell, and hearing, the nonspectacular senses. These grandest of animals cannot see very well. Is, then, the gaze of the dead big elephant looking up at the living little king, *witnessed* to in Derrida's counterfable, "the gaze of a seer, a visionary or extra-lucid blind one" that Derrida invokes in *The Animal that Therefore I Am*? Perhaps, as Derrida suggests in *Memoirs of the Blind*, the function of the eye is not to see, but to cry, like the tear-filled eye of the elephant mourning his kin. "The eye would be destined not to see but to weep. . . . The blindness that opens the eye is not the one that darkens vision. The revelatory or apocalyptic blindness, the blindness that reveals the very truth of the eyes, would be the gaze veiled by tears" (Derrida 1993, 126–27). Whether we mean the actual eye or the metaphorical mind's eye, only if we "see" vision or disclosure as the proper (and perhaps only) function of the eye do we see blindness or lack of vision (lack of the *as such*) as a defect. What if, instead, we take the purpose of the eye to be tears, crying for loved ones? Or crying tears of joy for sharing a life with other beloved creatures, a sharing that gives life meaning and opens onto a new love of life itself? These would be tears of compassion for all other living beings. Seeing as necessarily veiled in tears. Loving so much it hurts. If the eye is not for seeing but for crying, then elephants are superior to humans in their capacity for both kinship and mourning.

"If You Can't Be Good, Be Careful!"

In conclusion, we might ask, does deconstruction leave us with a way of imagining witnessing that is not autopsic, and sovereignty that does not require capital punishment? Indeed, can we "do" philosophy that is not also autopsy and that does not ground itself in death penalties? Insofar as philosophy itself is an assertion of judgment, decision, and sovereignty, the most capital of disciplines, how can we move beyond autopsic ways of seeing, and killing in the name of sovereignty? How can we think beyond cruel and unusual punishments when our very thinking, the ability to think, is bound to technologies of autopsy and death? How do we open ourselves to the uncanny otherness that comes uninvited? In other words, what is this passive activity of letting or waiting? Between witnessing as testifying to one's own trustworthiness or one's own sovereignty, and witnessing as bearing witness to something other, something beyond recognition, perhaps there is another way, a way to witness as bearing, rather than bearing witness. Rather than standing erect atop the ivory tower watching the world from a distance, as a spectator on high, in order to testify to what we see with our mind's eye, we bear witness in the sense of bringing forth. Rather than claiming philosophy as our inheritance, our birthright, or the product of our own making, our own sovereignty, we bear it in the sense of *parere*, or bringing forth, and *patere*, or lying open. We give up the fabulous illusion that we can control our own work, or that we give birth to ourselves through it.

Of his own work, Derrida says in his last interview, *Learning to Live Finally*:

> Each time, however faithful one might want to be, one ends up betraying the singularity of the other whom one is addressing. The same goes a fortiori when one writes books for a more general audience: you do not know to whom you

are speaking, you invent and create silhouettes, but in the end it no longer
belongs to you. Spoken or written, all these gestures leave us and begin to act
independently of us. Like machines, or better, like marionettes. . . . I become,
appearing-disappearing, like that uneducable specter who will have never
learned how to live. The trace I leave signifies to me at once my death,
either to come or already come upon me, and the hope that this trace
survives me. (2007, 32)

Learning to live, he says, is learning to die, which may be impossible. How
to die? Like eating and mourning, we all must "do" it, so the question is
how to do it well. Yet, like suffering, it is not really something we "do," but
rather something we undergo—something that happens to us, not something we make happen (even if we commit suicide). But if writing is dying,
then Derrida dies well. For him, however, writing or dying well is not a
matter of salvation or redemption. It is not for the sake of another life worth
more than this one that he writes or teaches. Yet he does write for "an
unforeseeable future-to-come," one that he attempts to conjure through
words (see 2004, 4). We seem to be between two futures, the unforeseeable
one and the one of absolute judgment and redemption. How to live for the
sake of the former without also invoking the later?

As we have seen, Derrida describes a difference between the "official"
aesthetics of political discourse or even of political philosophy and the
aesthetics of art or poetry. Indeed, he goes further to suggest that a political
revolution "worthy of its name" requires a poetic revolution. In other
words, what Julia Kristeva might call an imaginary revolt, or, we might say,
poetic revolution, requires a change in the way that we imagine ourselves,
others, and our relationships to the world. As we have seen, Kristeva goes
so far as to say that art and aesthetic experience are transformative, and, by
sublimating sadomasochistic impulses, can prevent violent acting out.

Although they use different terminology, at bottom, for both Derrida
and Kristeva, the majesty of poetry and art brings forth an encounter with
uncanny otherness, while the majesty of political sovereignty forecloses
otherness with its gestures of absolute mastery. Both tend toward hyperbolic and excessive gestures. But while poetry and art point to what
always remains in excess of any attempt at mastery, sovereignty claims
absolute control that leaves no remainder. In a sense, it is the difference
between, on the one hand, trying to control language by mastering it in
order to wield political power—the politician as master of rhetoric—and,

on the other, listening to language through disciplining oneself and letting language speak. Yet this difference may be only a hairsbreadth; and moreover, it may be impossible to tell which is which, which is precisely why we must keep trying, and why we must be careful.

Derrida refuses to merely take on the clichés like a machine, but at the same time, he listens to them. Rather than close himself off, deny the sensory dimension of language for the sake of mastering it, Derrida's masterful writing is a form of listening that he describes as a struggle with the French language, a hand-to-hand combat. He says that "my desire resembles that of a lover of the tradition who would like to free himself from conservatism. Imagine someone who is mad for the past . . . but a madman who dreads fixation on the past, nostalgia, the cult of remembrance. A contradictory and uncomfortable double injunction" (2004, 4). This double injunction requires that he/we take on the traditions that we inherit, but do so responsibly through "active intervention," through an active listening. He/we must listen to the point of losing our minds, losing our eyes and our "I"s.

Derrida teaches us that there is more than one way of losing your mind, or your eyes/I's. There is the way of sovereign mastery that denies that anything or anyone is out of reach, out of control, including one's own body. This way of losing the "I" is the way of disavowing that the "I" is merely a performance, an erection. In absolute terms, it is the operation of effacing the "I" of both the narrator necessary to testify to the performance and the "I" of the sovereign as an individual man like anyone else. It is the displacement of the eye for an eternal "I" that sees itself as lord and master over everything in its purview, which is to say everything. The other way of losing the "I," of losing one's mind, is through poetry or art, which is to say an encounter with uncanny otherness, even absurdity. Rather than cutting off any possibility of excess or remainder, this aesthetic rejoices in it.

Derrida describes the style of deconstruction as "a *jouissance* of the concept to the point of overflowing" (2004, 5). There is a pleasure in excess, a joy in being overtaken by it. He describes deconstruction as "hyperconceptual" insofar as "it carries out a large-scale consumption of concepts that it produces as much as it inherits—but only to the point where a certain writing, a writing that thinks, exceeds the conceptual 'take' and its mastery. It therefore attempts to think the limit of the concept; it even endures the experience of this excess; it lovingly lets itself be exceeded. It is like an ecstasy of the concept: a *jouissance* of the concept to the point of over-flowing" (2004, 5). He teaches us to enjoy the multiple, even contradictory, meanings, which exceed our control or mastery. Rather than dissect them and pin them down in the laboratory of philosophical autopsy for the sake of clear and distinct ideas or self-certainty, he accepts, even loves, the uncanny excess always out of control. This does not mean, however, that there are no rules, that anything goes, or that we can do whatever we like with the concepts we inherit or with our tradition.

We are always caught up in the machine. We are always like marionettes controlled by forces beyond us. Yet this does not mean that we are deter-mined and therefore absolved of responsibility. Again, this is the double injunction of deconstructive ethics. We are responsible even though we cannot control ourselves. We are ethically bound even though we cannot be certain of the difference between right and wrong. The imperative of deconstructive ethics puts us in this double bind: We have infinite ethical obligations precisely because we are infinite beings. Derrida says that only finite beings inherit; and this inheritance brings with it obligations both to the past and to the future: "Only a finite being inherits, and his finitude obliges him. It obligates him to receive what is larger and older and more powerful and more durable than he. But the same finitude obliges one to choose, to prefer, to sacrifice, to exclude, to let go and leave behind. Precisely in order to respond to the call that preceded him, to answer it and to answer for it—in one's name as in the name of the other" (2004, 5). The question, then, is again, how? How to answer in one's own name and in the name of the other?

How can we respond to the call from the other whom we may not recognize or hear? How can we be vigilant in our listening when we don't even know what we are listening for? How do we let ourselves be surprised? How do we avoid becoming mere "answering machines"? (see 2002a, 100). To have a ready-made answer to moral dilemmas or a set of rules of etiquette for every situation is to become like a machine that reacts rather than responds. Morality becomes a matter of plugging in the data and spitting out the answer. This is when morality becomes unethical. Yet there are rules. There is grammar. There are conventions. We do inherit. We use clichés. But neither the machinery of nature nor the machinery of culture that move us like so many marionettes absolves us of responsibility. Neither determinism nor constructivism enables us to escape the binding force of obligation. Moreover, Derrida refuses the very opposition between naturalism and constructivism because the meeting of these two machines always produces a remainder, something in excess of the rules.

Again, this is not to say that anything goes. Rather, Derrida insists that the undecidability necessary for response through which we may hope to avoid becoming mere answering machines is not a form of relativism. He may multiply meanings and interpretations, but always within the grammar of the language he inherits, even as he insists on an absolute untranslatabilty and the excess produced through that grammar (cf. 2009, 170, 302; 2002b). Discussing his position on sovereignty, he insists, "what I here call 'responsibility' is what dictates the decision to be sometimes *for* the sovereign state and sometimes *against* it, for its deconstruction ('theoretical and practical,' as one used to say) according to the singularity of the contexts and the stakes. There is no relativism in this, no renunciation of the injunction to 'think' and to deconstruct the heritage. This aporia is in truth the very condition of decision and responsibility—if there is any. . . . No one can make me respond to this question as though it were a matter of pressing a button on some old-fashioned machine" (2004, 92). Each time, each decision, requires thought, reflection, and response. But this is not the thought of some cogito that can ever get a clear and distinct idea free from all conditions. Still, it is a matter of distinguishing and discerning, of multiplying limits and borders rather than closing them down, of making more rather than less. But this making more also requires great care. Derrida repeatedly warns us to be careful, to go slowly, not to rush, not to become answering machines, which is easier said than done—if possible at all.

Whenever I left her, my grandmother used to say to me, "Be good, and if you can't be good, be careful." A version of this could be a motto for deconstructive ethics: "Be good, *and since you can't* be good, be careful." We try to discern good from evil, but since we can never be certain that we have done so, we must be vigilant. Ethics is not a one-time operation. Rather, it is a matter of infinite responsibility alive in finite beings. This is why responsibility is never far from death and mourning. If, as Nietzsche says, "all joy wants eternity," Derrida suggests that joy is possible only for finite beings; indeed, joy is always already dead, always past, always of yesterday and the passing of the present moment into the past: "I enjoy from yesterday . . . because only yesterday will have given me, only my death or the feeling of my death . . . only my death lets me enjoy and take pleasure—in this very moment. . . . Without mourning, and the mourning of myself, the mourning of my 'I am present,' there would be no pleasure" (2011, 53). Yet if we think that we can mourn once and for all, or that we can sublimate death or the death drive once and for all, then we risk giving it to our autopsic impulse and falling back into the deadly conceit of sovereign mastery over ourselves and over others.

SIX

Deadly Devices: Animals, Capital Punishment, and the Scope of Sovereignty

> Tennyson's agonizing line—"Nature red in tooth and claw"—tends, especially in these days of world-wide human carnage, to make one see the whole animal kingdom with blood-dripping claws and jaws. But it is not so. . . . Nature as seen in animal life is sanguinary, but only man is cruel.
>
> — JOHN BORROUGHS, *North American Review*, October 1918

Can animals be sentenced to death? Can they be assassinated, or become victims of genocide? Certainly in our common parlance, these dubious rights are reserved for man; murder, assassination, genocide, and the death penalty are proper to man alone. Even in death, we insist upon separating ourselves from the animals. Yet our practices suggest otherwise. Animals are regularly killed for "crimes" committed against humans. For example, recently in Switzerland a swan was killed for trying to drown a swimmer by sitting on him; and dogs are regularly "put down" if they are considered dangerous. Unlike humans, however, usually animals are not subjects of the law and therefore are not entitled to a fair trial. But, as we will see, this was not always the case.

In *For What Tomorrow*, Derrida describes the death penalty as the "weld" or "cement" that holds together Western traditions of religion, philosophy, and politics—in other words, everything that is taken to be "proper to man."

He concludes, "the death penalty would be the keystone . . . of the onto-theological-political . . . along with the nature-technique distinction and everything that follows from it . . . a properly and strictly human and supposedly rational law" (2004, 148). He suggests that what is taken to be properly and strictly human follows from the death penalty; and the division between man and animal at the heart of these traditions ultimately rests on the death penalty. Critically alluding to Martin Heidegger's claim that animals do not die but merely perish—a claim that Derrida has explicitly challenged in various texts—he says, "The death penalty would thus be, like death itself, what is 'proper to man' in the strict sense" (2004, 147).[1]

As we know, according to Heidegger and others, animals do not die, they merely perish (cf. Derrida 2009, 123). Supposedly because animals have no concept of death, they cannot die in the way that we do. Or, as medieval Christian theologians believed, animals have no soul, so they cannot live or die as we do. For Descartes animals are like machines, never really alive and therefore already dead. And, for Kant, they are not rational and therefore do not have or require the dignity that we do. In *The Animal that Therefore I Am*, Derrida challenges these views by suggesting, on the one hand, that we cannot be sure that animals do not possess these qualities, and on the other, that we cannot be sure that we do possess them. Following Derrida, we might ask in what sense *we* have a concept of death. More specifically, what would it mean to say that we are *conscious* of death? After all, who can give a first-hand account of the consciousness of death? How can we be sure that we die rather than merely perish, since death remains a mystery to us? Moreover, how can we be sure that we know better than other animals what it is to die, or to live, for that matter?

Taking on the traditional opposition between man and animal, particularly in terms of death and the death penalty, Derrida argues, "A 'deconstruction' of what is most hegemonic in philosophy should therefore include a deconstruction of the death penalty, and of everything with which it is in solidarity—beginning with a certain concept of sovereignty—of its entire scaffolding (*and likewise, of the discourse on what is called 'the animal'*)" (Derrida 2004, 88; my emphasis). What are we to make of this parenthetical remark about the discourse of "the animal"? How is "the animal" related to the death penalty, especially if the death penalty is reserved for man alone?

In this chapter, I want to explore the connections between speculation, spectacle, and the death penalty, particularly insofar as they bear on what is proper to man and on the man-animal distinction. I will analyze how "what is called the animal" shows up as a parenthesis in the history of the death penalty and of the sovereignty that it guarantees; man's dominion over other animals is built on a model of sovereignty that is built on the scaffolding of death and the death penalty. Following the history of the death penalty, we will see that it becomes the property of man through its exercise on animals, particularly through the capital punishment of animals that inaugurated the codification of law in modern Europe, on the one hand, and Thomas Edison's electrocution of animals that inaugurated use of the electric chair as a form of execution in the United States, on the other. Moreover, the case of Edison, who invented both the electric chair and the first moving pictures, many of which were images of executions, makes manifest the connection between spectacle, animals, and the death penalty. Analyzing the conjunction of cinematic spectacle and executions, I show how the notion of instant death or clean death is a fantasy. Moreover, examining early cinematic representations of execution, specifically the films of Edison, demonstrates how cuts, pans, and splices are necessary to create a convincing image of instant death. I argue that the current three-drug lethal injection, the only method of execution approved by the Supreme Court in the United States, includes within it a supplement that creates the look of death before actual death. In this way, as we will see, the fantasy of instant death is maintained and created through technological interventions whose history is intimately connected to animals.

Here, I trace an alternative genealogy of man's sovereignty through which he becomes morally and legally responsible by virtue of what we might call *animal experiments* within the penal code. These animal experiments eventually give way to our current considerations of animals as property, but only after establishing sovereignty as the property of man. Both civil law and various forms of punishment were tried on animals before they became the sole property of man. The transition from religious law to civil law involved extending legal codes to all of the animal kingdom in order to establish the sovereignty and dominion of civil law over all creatures. The death penalty was applied equally to man and beast. Man became a proper moral and legal subject through the exercise of the death penalty on animals. Animals played the contradictory role of shoring up the absolute authority of the law on the one hand, and eventually through their exclusion, shoring up man's membership in the moral and civil community on the other hand. In addition, as the case of Edison demonstrates, animals were not only the test subjects for the codification of Roman law, but also the test subjects for the punishments enacted by that law. Specifically, animals were instrumental in the invention of the electric chair, which ushered in the technological age of killing machines. In the end, I argue that the history of the death penalty undermines the notion that it is the property of man, and that the current protocol for lethal injection undermines our ability to answer questions of consciousness with certainty. The question of the consciousness of death is just as uncertain in humans as it is in animals.

Animal Executions: Establishing Man's Property and What Is Proper to Man

As we have seen, Derrida's discussion of the scale of sovereignty and its autopsic or scopic modalities revolves around a seventeenth-century elephant autopsy, wherein "[n]ever perhaps was there a more imposing anatomical dissection, judged by the enormity of the animal, by the precision with which its several parts were examined, or by the quality and number of those present" (2009, 250). This spectacle performs and establishes the king's sovereignty over both man and beast. While this elephant apparently died of natural causes, during this time throughout Europe, other animals were brought to trial and executed. From the Middle Ages through the seventeenth century, with the first codifications of law, punishment was exacted against man and beast alike to establish the scope of the law's sovereignty over all of creation. From the Middle Ages, France in particular levied capital punishment on animal offenders. Pigs, apparently criminal by nature, were frequent defendants in capital crimes and were often executed by hanging. For example, in 1457 in Savigny, a pig and her six piglets were caught "red-hoofed," so to speak, in the act of murder: "a pig and six suckling piglets . . . having been captured in flagranti since these pigs have committed and done themselves murder" of a five-year-old girl (Sorel 1876, quoted in Dinzelbacher 2002, 407). While the sow was sentenced to be hanged, the piglets, "in default of any positive proof that they had assisted in mangling the deceased, although covered with blood . . . were restored to their owner on the condition that he should give bail" ("Execution of Animals for Crimes" 1860, 2).

The first president of the French Parlement de Provence (something like Chief Justice) and "a significant contributor to the evolution of sixteenth-century French legal thought," Bartholomew Chassenée, became famous for defending animals at trial (see Girgen 2003, 101–02; cf. Evans 1906). The case that established him as an "eminent legal scholar" was a defense of the rats of Autun, who were going to lose by default for not appearing in court when summoned. Chassenée won the case, arguing that because his clients lived in different villages a single summons could not reach all of them, so they should be summoned individually; that the journey was too long; and that the rats feared the cats they would encounter on the way (see Girgen 2003, 102). In my survey of the literature on animal trials I found that, although some challenge his sources, most scholars agree with E. P. Evans's 1906 overview in *The Criminal Prosecution and Capital Punishment of Animals* that the practice of executing animals served at least to reestablish the supposed natural order wherein man ruled over animals and to establish the scope of the law across the entire animal kingdom. In other words, animals were subject to the newly codified law to establish the state's authority across the human and animal kingdoms.

Other rationales for capital punishment for animals include biblical sources that require an eye for an eye from animals as well as from man. Consider the famous passage Exodus 21:28: "If an ox gore a man or a woman, that they die; then the ox shall be surely stoned, and his flesh shall not be eaten," and 21:31: "Whether he have gored a son, or have gored a daughter, according to this judgment shall it be done to him" (here the pronoun is ambiguous and could mean that the owner shall pay his ransom or die with his ox). The biblical principle of *lex talionis*, or retaliation, was extended into Roman law, and throughout this period was practiced against man and animal alike.

Also, Leviticus 20:15–16 states that if a man or woman lies with a beast, both the human and the animal will be killed; and there are many cases of trials for bestiality in which the man and the beast were both executed for their crimes. Although bestiality accounted for 25 to 35 percent of all capital punishments in the seventeenth and eighteenth centuries in Sweden, and usually both man and beast were executed, in 1750, again in France, Jacques Ferron was caught in the act with a donkey. After much deliberation that included testimony from the parish priest as to the donkey's virtuous character and a signed document from members of the community

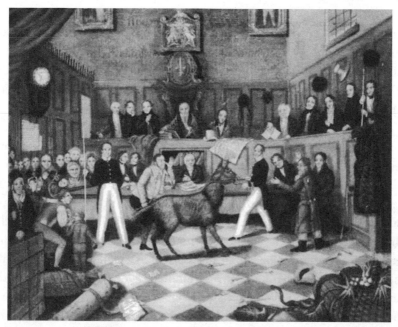

Charles Hunt after original by P. Mathews, "The Trial of Bill Burn Under Martin's Act." Second quarter of the nineteenth century but after August 1838. Contains Parliamentary information licensed under the Open Parliament Licence v1.0.

that the donkey was "a most honest creature," the court acquitted the donkey as a victim of the crime (see Seshadri-Crooks 2003, 11). As recently as the early twentieth century, in Kentucky and Tennessee animals were being tried and punished for bestiality (Girgen 2003, 122). As late as 1998, in Texas, a dog-bite victim selected a canine defendant from a doggie line-up (Girgen 2003, 123 fn183). And after pleas from celebrities including Bridget Bardot, another death-row dog, Taro, was "pardoned" by Governor Christine Todd Whitman as her seventh executive order after taking office, ending years of legal battles (Girgen 2003, 125). Technically Taro could not be pardoned because he is a dog, so Whitman remitted forfeiture of Taro as his owner's personal property.

While animals are still subject to the law and can be sentenced to death, their status as legal subjects is ambiguous. According to the letter of the law, they are merely property. But the ways in which they are dealt with by the courts suggests that their status is much more complicated, especially when malicious motives are attributed to them, or character witnesses attest to their criminal behavior as anomalous. In the case of Taro, thanks to Governor Whitman's executive order, the dog was merely exiled from New Jersey rather than killed. A *New York Times* headline read "The Dog Walks," while CNN ran "Death Row Dog Gets New Leash on Life" (Girgen 2003, 126).

One turn-of-the-century case of animal execution in Erwin, Tennessee stands out, given the enormity of its victim and the spectacle surrounding her hanging. On September 12, 1916, "Murderous Mary," as she came to be called—advertised as "The Largest Living Animal on Earth"—an Asian elephant who had been traveling with the Sparks Circus for twenty years, was arrested and taken to the county jail after she killed a novice handler who prodded her with a bull-hook behind the ear when she was reaching for a piece of watermelon along the side of the road. There was public outcry to kill the elephant, and it was rumored that a lynch mob was on the way, armed with a Confederate cannon (Dominey 2011). The problem was how to kill a four-ton elephant. The circus owner decided to hang Mary from a railroad crane. Reportedly, news traveled fast and thousands of people came out of the hills to watch Mary hang. On the first try, the chain broke, Mary fell, the crowd ran for fear of the murderous beast, and she had to be hanged again.

The only photo of the event is rumored to been the result of a request by the media that Mary be hanged a third time for a photo-op, and photography experts have apparently confirmed that the image has been retouched because visibility was low on that fateful foggy day in rural Tennessee; indeed, some even suggest that the elephant in the photograph may not be Mary, but a substitute (Dominey 2011). To complicate the metonymical circuit driven by our fascination with this enormous spectacle of execution, it has been reported "that some local residents recall 'two Negro keepers' being hung alongside Mary, and that others remember Mary's corpse being burned on a pile of crossties" (Schroeder 1997). According to folklorist Thomas Burton, "This belief may stem from a fusion of the hanging with another incident that occurred in Erwin, the burning on a pile of crossties of a Negro who allegedly abducted a white girl" (Burton 2004, 224). The Shroeder article concludes: "The murder of an elephant: a spectacle. The murder of 'a Negro': another spectacle" (Schroeder 1997). The history of execution, and of the death penalty, is one of spectacle, where entire

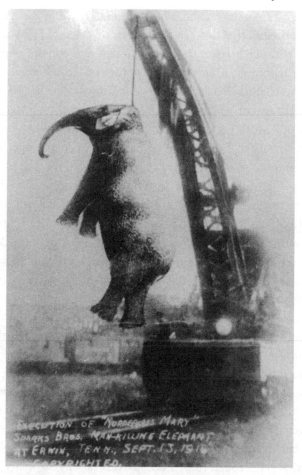

Execution of "Murderous Mary." (Appalachian Photographic Archive, Archives of Appalachia, East Tennessee State University, Johnson City, Tennessee.)

families watched lynching and hangings and photographed them as records of their outing.

Executing an Elephant

On January 4th, 1903, another elephant was executed, this time by the famous inventor Thomas Edison, who electrocuted the elephant Topsy, a Coney Island circus attraction who had killed three of her trainers, after one of them tried to feed her a lighted cigarette. We could say that because she wouldn't smoke a cigarette like a human and for the amusement of humans, she had to die. (Or, as Elissa Marder put it in her comments on a version of this chapter: Because she wouldn't smoke, she had to fry.) Edison documented the event, which was also a public spectacle reportedly attended by 1,500 people, with his short film entitled *Electrocuting an Elephant*. Just over a decade earlier, Edison had invented the Kinetoscope, a peephole device that allowed viewers to watch simple short films. The elephant film brought together Edison's most significant inventions, electric lighting, film, and electrocution as a means of administering the death penalty. The film was also a publicity stunt on the part of Edison, who waged what he called a "war of currents" with his rival George Westinghouse. Edison had invested in direct current (DC) electricity while Westinghouse had invested in alternating current (AC), which could be more easily transmitted at higher voltages over cheaper wires. In a campaign to discredit alternating current, Edison tried to convince people that it wasn't safe, first by using it to electrocute animals and eventually by endorsing it for use in executing humans. Edison reasoned that people would not want the same current flowing into their homes that was used for the electric chair.

Discussing Edison's cinematic executions, some of which were part of his campaign against Westinghouse, film critic Mary Ann Doane suggests, "Just as electricity could be activated as a technological control over life and death, the cinema must have seemed to offer the same promise in the field of representation" (2002, 164). Perhaps this is why so many early films feature executions, whether real executions of animals or reenacted executions of humans (or in Jean Renoir's 1939 *Rules of the Game*, both; see Sobchack 1984, 293). The hope was that if film could capture the moment of death, then it would unlock the secrets of life. But the slow process of a natural death is not what viewers want to see, not just because of mores that frown upon images of death and dead (human) bodies, but also because a natural death would take too long and risk losing its value as cinematic spectacle. Viewers want to see *instant death*, the kind that only execution could guarantee. But as analysis of the early images of executions show, the transition from animate to inanimate is not enough to convince spectators that they are witnessing real death or the instant of death. Indeed, in many cases of death, there may be little noticeable change in bodily movement without close inspection of breath or pulse. The fantasy of instant death could only be enacted via supplements, including not only showing the killing apparatus itself, but moreover offering visual and narrative representations of such a death. More precisely, these visual and narrative representations create the illusion of instant death through cuts, edits, and framing, or what we might call the *scaffolding* of death and the death penalty. It is the cuts, edits, frames, and scaffolding that are not seen, indeed that are necessarily hidden, which create the effect of instant death.

Edison's early film *Electrocuting an Elephant* promised to show viewers not only the deadly power of AC electricity but also the transition from life to death, something that paintings and photographs could not do. It promised to reveal the instant, the moment, or the truth, of death (cf. Combs 2008). In addition to the inherent connection between cinema and the scopic impulse to look, the birth of cinema makes manifest the intimate connection between film and the autopsic model of sovereignty and power, most especially man's dominion over animals and our own animal bodies. For the very first moving images were used in the service of scientific knowledge in laboratories and explicitly aimed at revealing life—animal life—in motion. The scientific films of Marey in France and Muybridge in the United States were some of the first moving images; and not coincidently, they involved animals, specifically frogs, dogs, and horses (see Cartwright 1992). These early films were *living autopsies* of sorts that revealed the workings of living bodies, animal bodies, as they underwent various surgeries and experiments. They were "spectacles of life and death" that fascinated scientists and the general public. As film historian Lisa Cartwright concludes, "More than documenting the elephant's death, [Edison's] one-minute *Electrocuting an Elephant* documents the technological implementation of a life and death process. As part of the overall experimental apparatus, the cinema apparatus both calibrates and helps determine what is it that constitutes life" (1992, 149)—and, we might add, death. Technologies of death produce the meaning of death through the image of death as framed, edited, narrated, contextualized, and in the case of Edison, even patented and marketed.

Edison reportedly executed so many stray cats and dogs, often in circus-like spectacles involving first shocking the animals with direct current and then killing them instantly with alternating current, that the area near his lab in Menlo Park, New Jersey was almost devoid of strays. In 1887, he held a public demonstration in West Orange, New Jersey, where he used a Westinghouse generator to kill a dozen animals at once, which spurred the media to use a new term to describe death by electricity, "electrocution" (Bellis 2011). A year later, Edison hired Harold Brown to help design the electric chair that would be used in the first execution of a prisoner, William Kemmler, by electrocution, which Edison called "being Westinghoused" (Bellis 2011). Brown continued Edison's experiments on animals, electrocuting strays, along with larger animals such as cows and horses. The day before the first use of the electric chair on a human, Brown tested 1000 volts on a horse, which was killed immediately. This test was conducted to establish how much AC electricity should be used on Kemmler. Reportedly, after 17 seconds of 1000 volts, Kemmler was pronounced dead by the attending physician. But after a member of the gallery pointed out that he was still breathing, the doctor quickly ordered another jolt of 2000 volts. "According to witnesses, the second jolt caused his blood vessels to burst and his skin to catch fire"; and a *New York Herald* correspondent described the execution: "'The scene of Kemmler's execution was too horrible to picture. He died the death of Feeks, the lineman, who was slowly roasted to death in the sight of thousands'" (Long 2008). George Westinghouse, who refused to sell his AC equipment for electrocution purposes, and who paid the legal fees for death row prisoners to appeal the death sentence, reportedly remarked, "They would have done better using an ax," the instrument that the jealous Kemmler had used to kill his wife after an argument (Long 2008).

Another eyewitness pointed to the difficulty of determining death by electrocution: "For obvious reasons, the only means of determining the question of death while the body was in circuit was by ocular monstration; so that it can not be positively asserted that the heart's action entirely ceased with the onset of unconsciousness" (physician Carlos MacDonald, quoted in Combs 2008). This raises the question of how to interpret or "read" the evidence of death—or loss of consciousness—from outside the victim's body (cf. Combs 2008). This question is not unique to electrocution, but rather raises more general questions: What counts as death? Is death instantaneous? And what is the relationship between dying and death? Doesn't the fantasy of instant death—the flipping of a switch, the push of a plunger— disavow not only the process of death but also whatever relationship death has to time and to our own finitude?

Even after the horrific report of Kemmler's execution, most eastern and southern states adopted the electric chair as the most humane method of execution, one that came to be known as "riding the lightning." With courts and prisons seemingly disavowing the grisly effects of electrocution, and holding on to the fantasy of instant death through electricity, the electric chair remained in use in the United States from 1890 through March 2010. After 1982, however, lethal injection replaced electrocution as the form of capital punishment considered most "humane." Until recently, the standard protocol for lethal injection, and still the only one approved by the Supreme Court, involved three drugs: the first rendering the prisoner unconscious, the second paralyzing the muscles, and the third stopping the heart. The Court ruled that as long as the condemned is unconscious at the time of death, then the punishment is not "cruel and unusual." Yet consciousness, or unconsciousness, is always in excess of what can be witnessed. What would it mean to say that we see or witness consciousness, or the lack of it? One of the drugs in the court-approved three-drug "cocktail" used for lethal injections, however, is no longer being made, and states have had to halt executions because they don't have legally sanctioned means to carry them out. The shortage of sodium thiopental, the anesthetic that renders prisoners unconscious, has done more to stop implementation of the death penalty in the United States than centuries of protests. States such as Tennessee that have tried to use suppliers not approved by the FDA have had their supplies of the drug seized by the federal government; in Tennessee 86 prisoners are now waiting on death row for execution. In addition, attorneys for several Tennessee death-row inmates have successfully challenged the state's method of determining whether inmates are unconscious before being put to death; rendering the condemned unconscious was the purpose of the discontinued drug (Haas 2011). It is noteworthy for my purposes that many states are now considering using one injection of pentobarbital, the drug most commonly used by veterinarians to euthanize animals. In fact, this was the drug used in the recent executions of Troy Davis in Georgia and Lawrence Brewer in Texas.

The second supplementary injection (supplementary to inducing unconsciousness, and to stopping the heart) makes the condemned appear unconscious, whether he is or not. It paralyzes his muscles, so that he cannot display or communicate either consciousness or pain. This injection can only be for the sake of the witnesses, who want to see an inert body devoid of movement, unlike the wracked and bleeding bodies aflame in the electric chair, or the twitching bodies of electrocuted animals. The second injection, then, completes the state's disavowal of the process of dying by rendering the prisoner motionless before the moment of death. Commenting on the "purifying" effect of lethal injection, Derrida says, "this disavowal of death, a way of denying it while imposing it . . . consists in making sure that there is nothing visible: no blood, no suffering" (2004, 136). This "clean death," sterilized with high-tech medical apparatus, including IVs, syringes, and hospital gurneys, supposedly sanitizes death; and like the "surgical strike" in high-tech warfare, it focuses death into an imagined instant, but only by dividing the process into the three stages of lethal injection that insure that the prisoner will look dead before he actually is dead. The look of death, then, is a necessary supplement to the real thing. Moreover, the look of death itself is created through a supplement to the visual space, a cut, an edit, a second injection that produces the look of death as part of our fantasy that death has a present and an instant.

But what does death look like? What do we see—or want to see—when we look at death? Like early films of execution and death, these high-tech executions create the illusion of death as a necessary supplement to the real thing. And it is telling that a prison's so-called theater of death resembles a movie theater! In addition, prisons have nurses and guards and an elaborate protocol for confirming that death has actually occurred. First the body is made to look dead, and then its death is confirmed by outside observers. Authentic first-hand testimony is not possible in the case of death. Given that no one can give first-hand testimony to the experience of death, we rely on witnesses, including doctors and scientists, and of course the performance of autopsy. Executions were once a form of public entertainment, and they still peak to our desire to witness death, which takes us back to Derrida's analysis of the autopsic impulse as part of the spectacle of power, power over animals, over the criminal elements in society, and over life and death themselves. Yet, insofar as death (and life) always exceeds the autopsic gaze, death operates as a limit event that makes manifest what Derrida identifies as the paradox of testimony in *The Instant of My Death/Demeure*: "When I testify, I am unique and irreplaceable. And at the very tip of this irreplaceability, this unicity, once again, there is the instant. Even if we have been several to participate in an event, to have been present at a scene, the witness can only testify when he asserts that he was in a unique place and where he could testify to this and that in a here-now, that is, in a pointed instant that precisely supports this exemplarity. The example is not substitutable; but at the same time the same aporia always remains: this irreplaceability must be exemplary, that is, replaceable. The irreplaceable must allow itself to be replaced on the spot. . . . The singular must be universalizable; this is the testimonial condition" (Derrida 2000, 41). The condition of the possibility of testimony—its uniqueness and irreplaceability—is destroyed by the act of testimony itself (cf. 2000, 33).

So, what would it be to witness to death? Given that no one has or can testify to his or her own death, it always requires external witnesses there at the scene. But, even then, that testimony is always a supplement to, and substitute for, the moment of death itself, which cannot be known or seen. And, as such, it operates as a disavowal of the fact the death is always beyond sovereignty, beyond knowledge, beyond the visual realm upon which we rely to confirm its existence. The same could be said of consciousness, which necessarily troubles the fantasy of instant, "clean" death imagined in the latest death penalty protocols involving lethal injection as a humane way to kill.

The paradox of witnessing is perhaps most obvious in the case of witnessing death, made evident in early execution films. Testimony becomes a necessary supplement to the truth of death, which cannot be seen in itself. Authentic death is produced through technologies of representation that augment the real event of death and make the image of death more real than death itself, precisely through its reproduction. The rupture between merely recording and representing an event is both literally and metaphorically sutured by cinematic editing techniques such that the "real" effect of death is created through cuts, fades, pans, and splices (cf. Sobchack 1984, Doane 2002, and Combs 2008). In an article entitled "Cut: Execution, Editing, and Instant Death," analyzing Edison's 1895 film *Execution of Mary, Queen of Scots*, film theorist Scott Combs says, "At Menlo Park in the 1880s, scientists and amateurs had divined the necessary charge of electrical current that would produce instantaneous death. Where animals did not die fast enough, they underwent a veritable process of torture. . . . Following on the heels of those experiments, the early films sought the quick fix—through beheading, hanging, electrocution, and other execution techniques—to inculcate the impression that the moving image camera could capture the change between life and death" (Combs 2008, 31). But as Combs argues, a dead or lifeless body is not enough to convince spectators of the veracity of death. Indeed, in order to appear lifelike, so to speak, not only is death doctored through cinematic techniques, but also it requires visual supplements that confirm that it has happened. The film itself is such a document, a supposed testament to a real event, a unique happening, only now framed and repeated as spectacle.

What counts as authentic death, then, is produced through technologies of representation that augment the real event of death and make the image of death more real than death itself, precisely through its reproduction (cf. Sobchack 1984, Doane 2002, and Combs 2008). Indeed, in order to appear lifelike, so to speak, not only is death doctored through cinematic techniques such as fades, cuts and pans, but also it requires visual supplements that confirm that it has happened. The film itself is such a document, a supposed testament to a real event, a unique happening, only now framed and repeated as spectacle.

A closer examination of three of Edison's execution films, *Electrocuting an Elephant*, *Execution of Mary, Queen of Scots*, and *Execution of Czolgosz*, shows the supplement necessary to create the spectacle of death, or simply put, the look of death. Although the first is a film of a real execution of an animal and the other two substitute dummies for human actors in reenactments, all three supplement the scene of death through editing and third-party confirmations. These images of death were not sufficient in themselves, but required supplemental narratives both within the films and accompanying the films, often in the form of lecturers who traveled with the films to explain and further frame what the spectator was to see in them. This was especially true of the early animal execution films, designed to warn of the dangers of AC electricity. In general, what the cuts, splices, substitutions, and narrative supplements suggest is that the image of death itself is not enough to establish its truth (cf. Doane 2002, 160).

For example, *Electrocuting an Elephant* (1903) does not reveal the instant of death or death as an instant, but rather executes death, such that, in the words of Doane, "*Electrocuting an Elephant* does not bring to its spectator the moment of death but its image, its sign, underscored by the film's inscription of lost time" (2002, 163–64). There is a cut in the middle of the film where it is obvious that the camera was stopped and then started again, leaving out the "lost time" of attaching the electrical apparatus, including wooden sandals attached to wires, to the elephant. "The event may take time, but it is packaged as a moment. . . . In *Electrocuting an Elephant*, time is certainly condensed and abstracted, but it also bears the stamp of an authenticity that is derived from the technological capabilities of the camera" (Doane 2002, 160). The film ends with a man entering the scene as if to confirm the elephant's death and the authenticity of the spectacle. Complicating Doane's analysis, I would add that the effect of the cut is paradoxical in that it both establishes the truth of the event while simultaneously undermining it. That is to say, the cut creates the illusion of two elephants—the live one walking along the train, and the rigid "dummy" elephant with smoke billowing from its feet. For a contemporary audience familiar with the simulacrum of authenticity created by cinema, the film is "watchable" only because the cut allows us, on some level, to disavow the real elephant's horrible death through the juxtaposition of the walking elephant and the rigid one. To speak tongue in cheek, perhaps given the shortage of lethal injection drugs, on the basis of the principle of *lex talionis*, or an eye for an eye, and in the name of the elephants harmed in the making of the electric chair, the United States should return to the ancient Asian

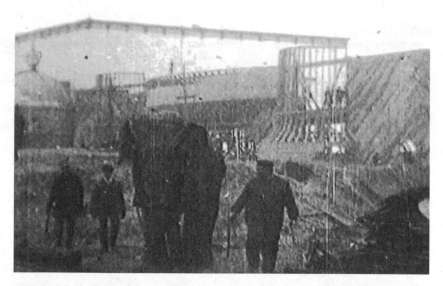

Still from "Electrocuting an Elephant" (film by Thomas Edison, 12 January 1903). (U.S. Dept. of Interior. National Park Service. Thomas Edison National Historical Park.)

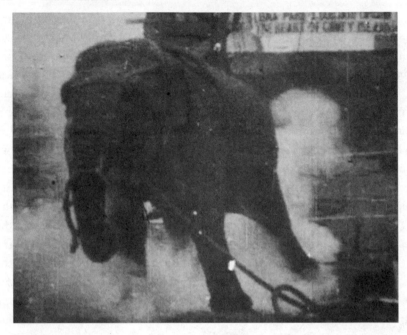

Still from "Electrocuting an Elephant" (film by Thomas Edison, 12 January 1903). (U.S. Dept. of Interior. National Park Service. Thomas Edison National Historical Park.)

practice of using elephants as our mode of execution, whereby an elephant is used to crush the condemned man.

For *Execution of Czolgosz* (1901), Edison could not get permission to film the actual execution of the prisoner, so he filmed the Auburn Prison on the day of the execution and substituted a reenactment for the execution itself. Here again, however, the viewer must be told that this prison is the very one where the execution is taking place, and that it is being filmed on the very day that execution is to happen. Not only does the spectacle of death require a substitution (obviously no actor will go that far for realistic effect!), but also it requires narrative supplements both internal to the film—panning the Auburn Prison, confirmation of electrocution by actors after the reenactment—and external to the film—knowledge that this is the very prison on the very day of the execution. Doane remarks on the "elaborate development of structures that produce the image of a coherent and unified 'real time' that is much more 'real' than 'real time' itself" (2002, 163).

In *Execution of Mary, Queen of Scots* (1895), again a dummy is substituted for the actor, and the scene is rendered nearly seamless through effective cutting and splicing. Adding another layer of substitution, Mary is played by a man dressed as a woman. And, as if the visual tricks of editing and substitution were not enough in themselves to convince the spectator that he or she had seen death, the last frame has the executioner holding up the (fake) head of the beheaded Mary, displaying it to the witnesses internal to the film as well as to the audience, as if to confirm death (cf. Combs 2008). Seeing an inert body, even a severed head, is not enough to convince us that death has occurred. Rather, we need confirmation by external witnesses who step in to check vital signs and tell us, Yes, he is dead (cf. Combs 2008, 32–34). Combs concludes, "The particular form of instantaneity assumed by the earliest recorded deaths could only be accommodated through supplemental features of stillness, gestures, and recognition outside the body in question" (34). And, since without editing, cutting, and splicing, "death is notoriously difficult to perceive . . . the duration of the shot undercuts the effect of the switch-like instant as measured as a slice of death," and thereby, "Film [both] replicates and annihilates instant death in the same move" (39).

The same could be said for the scientific quest for more humane capital punishment as a perverse enactment of the fantasy of instant death . . . or the development of smart bombs and surgical strikes that supposedly target only military outposts and personnel without killing civilians. For as we know, high-tech weaponry does not ensure that civilians, including animals and children, are not killed. Certainly the number of botched hangings, electrocutions, and lethal injections suggest that science cannot ensure instant death or that the victim is unconscious at the time of death. Execution by today's standard tripartite lethal injection merely produces the illusion or image of instant death, as if to ensure that what we believe we *witness* will be an instant death, even if the condemned is not actually dead yet. Furthermore, the supplemental confirmation of death by expert witnesses always comes too late to ensure instant death.

The most recent challenges to the death penalty have been attempts to apply the Eighteenth Amendment prohibiting cruel and unusual punishment, not just in terms of *lex talionis*, or retributions equal to the crimes committed, but also in terms of the mode of execution. In 2008 the Nebraska Supreme Court ruled electrocution cruel and unusual punishment after the hood worn by an inmate being executed caught fire and he continued breathing for minutes afterwards. Also in 2008, by a vote of 7 to 2, the U.S. Supreme Court upheld the use of lethal injection as a humane method of execution. The court's majority opinion suggests that if the prisoner is unconscious at the time of death, and if a strict medical procedure is followed, then inmates don't unduly suffer when executed. Leaving aside any emotional or psychological suffering, the court's ruling suggests that as long as there is no blood or fire, no outward or visible signs of the loss of bodily integrity, no bodily mess, then the punishment is not cruel. Scientific, medical, and technological intervention has been crucial in the court's upholding lethal injection as a humane mode of execution. Furthermore, we could say that the *technology* of death has been the machine with which the process or pain of dying has been disavowed. We hold on to a fantasy of a technologically mediated "clean" death that assumes not only that we know and can recognize the moment of death, but also and moreover that we can know and recognize the presence of consciousness; in other words, that both can be "seen" by external witnesses.

The preference for technologically mediated death, particularly high-tech executions involving machines that administer carefully measured lethal drugs at regulated intervals, takes us back to the opposition between nature and technology with which we began. Like high-tech weaponry used by industrial nations, high-tech death penalties of all sorts create the illusion of a clean or good death. As long as technologies of death promise immediate and instant death, they are not *seen* as cruel and unusual. Writing for the majority in the decision upholding lethal injection, Chief Justice Roberts contends that the state has adequately proved that the second injection that paralyzes the prisoner "serves two purposes: (1) preventing involuntary convulsions or seizures during unconsciousness, thereby preserving the procedure's dignity, and (2) hastening death" (*Baze vs. Rees* 2008). Yet the preservation of dignity and quick death can be ensured only if the body is made to look dead before it is dead. The scene of a clean or good death disavows the actual process of dying, which could be messy and bloody; in other words, death is always "in the eye of the beholder." Or, more accurately, the fantasy of death (or consciousness) is always in the eye of the beholder, a fantasy that is always haunted by powerlessness in the face of death and our inability to comprehend what it is . . . or what it looks like.

With the current three-drug protocol, we circumvent the questions of both "what is death?" and "what is consciousness?" by paralyzing the condemned such that both questions ultimately become irrelevant, at least to the courts and the prison systems administering it, as long as we cannot see suffering. Yet the supplement of the second, muscle-paralyzing drug ensures that we cannot see suffering, which is the very criterion for humane death that meets the standards against cruel and unusual punishment. In other words, the three-drug protocol makes it impossible to establish whether or not the condemned is suffering, and therefore whether or not his death is cruel. This fabulous disavowal of both the processes of consciousness (not to mention the unconscious) and of death evacuates the condemned man of the very keystone of phenomenology, the "consciousness of." Moreover, it disables any possibility of sovereignty in the sense of an "I can," insofar as it literally paralyzes him and leaves him not only facing execution but also life without *parole*, without speech, without any way to signal or express either his consciousness or his suffering. The question, then, of whether a punishment *is* cruel and unusual has been displaced onto the question of whether it *appears* to be cruel and unusual.

In *For What Tomorrow*, Derrida reminds us that the word *cruel* comes from the Latin root *crudus*, which means rough, raw, or bloody, and shares its root with the word *crude*. The crude or cruel death is one that is raw and bloody, not sterile and clean. Technology renders death "cooked"—sometimes even fried—rather than raw, bloody, and crude. *Crude* is defined as "in the natural and raw state, not changed by any process, preparation or manufacture" (*OED*). Cruelty is associated with the crude state of nature, specifically brutes, savages, and animals, which are seen as "red in tooth and claw." Tennyson's phrase, listed among synonyms for *cruelty* in Webster's, describes the cruelty of nature, particularly of predators who eat their prey raw and bloody. *Cruel*, then, is associated with nature and animals—red in tooth and claw—while *humane* is associated with technologically mediated, sterile, and bloodless death. The nature-culture opposition, "deconstructed" throughout Derrida's work from beginning to end, is now, and perhaps always was, put into the service of the death penalty. We imagine humane death as the clean, sterile death administered by high-tech machines and synthetically produced pharmaceuticals that feed our fantasy of instant death as painless death, because we do not see any signs of suffering.

Unlike other predatory beasts, with the help of technology we disavow our own cruelty, our own animality, and with it the nature of dying, whatever that might be. As long as we maintain the fantasy of bloodless, instant death, promised by technologies that make it as easy as flipping a switch, pushing the plunger, or pulling the plug, we maintain the reason for our commitment to a more humane death penalty, upon which our fabled humanity depends. The same could be said for high-tech death penalties of all sorts. Whether through capital punishment or high-tech warfare, we imagine that our technology purifies or annuls our own animality. We imagine that it is what separates us from other animals. And ultimately technology is what reassures us that our killing is not cruel because it is not crude. We hold fast to the fantasy that while other animals kill with bloodlust and cruelty, our high-tech killing offers bloodless, clean, and sterilized death, that is, death with dignity, the dignity that Immanuel Kant claimed distinguished us from animals.

As we have seen, however, technologies of death, including capital punishment, were first tried on animals. And the history of our justifications for humane death, whether of humans or of animals, is built on the scaffolding that brought countless animals to the gallows, whether literally or in laboratories, factory farms, or slaughterhouses. Our notion that death is proper to humans, that man alone is conscious of death, is undone from both sides. On the one hand, the history of the death penalty, supposedly proper to man, is irrevocably tied to the deaths of animals, whether those executed to legitimate the sovereignty of civil law or those who became the victims of Edison's vicious electrocutions that led to the invention of the electric chair. And, on the other hand, capital punishment as carried out in the United States operates to ensure that we circumvent the impossible question of the human consciousness of death through the second injection that paralyzes the muscles of the condemned.

In sum, we justify our uniquely human position in relation to death and all forms of death penalties, from capital punishment to war, by using and excluding animals and animality. These animals occupy an ambivalent place in the history of our legal system: on the one hand, just as responsible, just as guilty or innocent as any human; and on the other hand, supposedly without knowledge or consciousness of death. But what counts as knowledge or consciousness of death? And how can be we so sure we possess it and they do not? How do men die? And women? How do animals die?

And what of the various forms of killing, or of letting die, or of putting to sleep? What remains of the animal in our own remains? Once we begin to ask these questions, death and the death penalty as proper to man, as his property, appear as illusions, sleights of reason, with which we justify man's dominion over other animals.

And then more questions arise: Is it possible to perform an autopsy on an animal? Or are animals only the object of dissections or necropsy? What is a corpse, especially the corpse of an animal? Is it a body, an object, or a person? In the case of animals, can we even talk about corpses? Or, when they die, do they become mere carcasses (or dinner)?[2] Today, can animals be sentenced to death? Can they be assassinated, or become victims of genocide?[3] J. M. Coetzee's novel *Elizabeth Costello* raises these kinds of controversial questions when the title character compares the slaughter of animals for food to the slaughter of Jews in the Holocaust. Like other characters in the novel, some people are offended at the comparison—that Jews might be compared to animals, or that animals might be compared to people. In our common parlance, today these rights are reserved for man; murder, assassination, and genocide are proper to man alone. Only man can be the victim of crimes against humanity. Yet as we have seen, the history of sovereignty in relation to capital punishment suggests otherwise.

The stakes of my project come together at this point: from the machinations of deconstructive ethics as the dismantling of the scaffolding of sovereignty, to the erection of that scaffolding through the machinations of life and death authorized by the performance itself, through the appeals to theology that once again take us back to the animal, to the beast and the sovereign, between two marionettes. Sovereignty requires death and always erects itself by threatening death. Moreover, the death it requires is always the death of the animal, whether that so-called animal is a person deemed criminal, traitor, terrorist, or enemy, or is another living being deemed trophy, nuisance, dinner, or scientific experiment. And these distinctions between kinds of life and kinds of death take us back to fundamental oppositions presupposed between nature and technology, nature and law, and nature and culture. Once again, the nature-culture opposition is at the bottom of so many others, most especially the opposition between animal and man, which becomes the justification for violence against animals and man alike.

SEVEN

Death Penalties: Ethics, Politics, and the Unconscious of Sovereignty

Insofar as Western philosophy, like Christianity, begins with a scene of capital punishment—that of Socrates being sentenced and put to death— doesn't it also have its beginnings in the death penalty? Derrida answers that philosophers from Kant to Levinas justify the death penalty and "just" wars on the basis of *lex talionis*, which takes us back not only to its theological roots but also to the basis of sovereignty (2004, 146).[1] For the sake of protection by the state, citizens subject themselves to state sovereignty and grant to the state, and only to the state, the power to kill. In other words, all justified killing, killing that is not a crime, must be circumscribed by law, as in war or state-sanctioned execution. This is why for Kant it is better that the sovereign head of state be assassinated rather than be executed by law, since execution of the sovereign who makes and enforces the law would undermine the power of law itself (Kant 1996, 132).

Derrida claims that no philosopher *qua* philosopher has opposed the death penalty on principle, that from Plato through Heidegger, "each in his own way, and sometimes not without much hand-wringing (Rousseau), took a stand for the death penalty" (2004, 146). As we have seen, he concludes that the death penalty is the *keystone* of speculative philosophy, that the death penalty and sovereignty are built on the same scaffolding, and that the death penalty is the "weld" or "cement"—we might say *the bind, even the double bind*—"that holds together Western traditions of religion, philosophy, and politics" (2004, 88). Is it possible, then, to salvage notions of obligation and responsibility from both their Judeo-Christian heritage and their Enlightenment reincarnations, which not only reduce morality to a matter of calculation, accounting, and bookkeeping but also and moreover are built upon the scaffolding of *lex talionis*, which necessarily leads to the death penalty? Can we think ethics, or politics for that matter, beyond debt management, wherein taking a life, or more precisely, giving death, is the ultimate payback?

In this chapter, I take up these questions through an analysis of the tension between ethics and politics as it is articulated by Kant, Levinas, and Derrida in order to delineate both the ethical and political stakes in technologies of death. Beginning with Kant's notion of duty, or *Pflicht*, I argue that within this ethical concept there is already embedded a polis that takes us closer to contemporary continental thinkers such as Levinas and Derrida. Next, I turn to the centerpiece of hyperbolic ethics, the notion of responsibility, to show how it also already contains within it a polis. The tension between the unconditional and the conditional described by Derrida becomes the tension between the ethical and the political. This tension becomes more concrete when we examine the death penalty as it is exercised in the United States—and in particular, the recent protests against executing an allegedly innocent black man, Troy Davis. In the end, I argue that we need a psychoanalytic supplement to hyperbolic ethics in order to understand our own investments in state-sanctioned violence, whether we are for or against the death penalty. To begin to think about our own investments in state-sanctioned violence, we need to consider the ways in which death penalties of all kinds find their place not only in economic and political power struggles but also in the revenge fantasies that fuel them, whichever side they are on.

Ethics or *Politics: Kant and Levinas*

Since Kant, ethics has been synonymous with moral law, grounded in reason. As Kant's heirs, we are still grappling with a tension he sought to resolve through his appeal to a rational God, namely, between ethics and politics. "Politics says, 'Be ye wise as serpents,'" remarks Kant; "Morality adds (as a limiting condition) 'and guileless as doves'" (1996a, 338). For Kant, both the serpent of politics and the dove of ethics are bound by the same moral duty that has its source in the freedom of our sovereign rational will. The perfection of this good will is possible not on the level of individuals but only from the perspective of what Kant referred to, in the title of one of his essays, as "Universal History from a Cosmopolitan Point of View," which it turns out is a view from the cosmos, or more specifically, from the perspective of the "dwellers from other planets" whom Kant imagines viewing us from their own place in the universe (1963, n. 2).

As we know, Kant insists that the *concept* of duty cannot be in conflict with *doing* our duty—or, that *ought* implies *can*: "It is patently absurd, having granted this concept of duty its authority, to want to say that one nevertheless cannot do it. For in that case this concept would of itself drop out of morals. . . . [H]ence, there can be no conflict of politics as doctrine of right put into practice, with morals, as theoretical doctrine of right" (1996a, 338). But what if the reverse were true? What if *ought* implies *cannot*? What if our obligations always outstrip our intentions? What if the sovereign will is fundamentally beholden both to other people and to the Other of language and culture, such that Kant's autonomous "I can" becomes "I suffer"? In other words, what if in order to save the ethical import of the concept of duty, morality itself must drop out?

I am alluding to Levinas's notion of ethics as first philosophy, with all of the responsibility of modern ethics but none of its autonomy or self-certainty. Indeed, moving from Kant to Levinas, we could say that autonomy and responsibility become inversely proportioned. For as rational law, and self-sovereignty, and everything that grounds modern morality slip away, our ethical responsibility increases. As we shake the ground from our soles/souls as so much dirt stuck there, as Deleuze (1968, 197) might say, and give up our illusions of putting ourselves into the shoes of others, nonetheless, we still have one more step to take, one more response to give. As we move from Kant's moral law to Levinas's ethical insomnia, responsibility becomes ratcheted up to such a degree that Derrida calls it "hyperbolic ethics" (2001).

At first blush, it seems that all that Kant's duty and Levinas's responsibility have in common is the appeal to God, and even that is radically different between the two. It is noteworthy, however, that Kant's concept of duty, or *Pflicht*, could have been more literally translated as "plight" or even "pledge." Indeed the English word *plight* has its origins in the Old German word *Pflicht*. And *Pflichten* can be translated as "obligation" or "responsibility." Although I cannot follow the complex etymological connections that lead from *Pflicht* to *responsibility*, there are some forceful currents running through them, from the familiar connotations of obligation, promise, and binding to the extraordinary connotations of risk, danger, and hostage. The history of the words *Pflicht* and *Pflichten*, *plight*, *pledge*, and *responsibility* are bound together as they weave their way between German, French, and English, along with Old Dutch and their Latin roots. *Plight* means, among other things, to risk making oneself responsible for another, to pledge, to promise or warrant on another's behalf. A *pledge* is both a solemn oath and a person who becomes hostage or bail for another. And the Latin root of *responsibility*, *spondeo*, means to promise or warrant or to pledge, again both in the sense of vowing and of putting oneself up as bail or security for another. Both *plight* and *responsibility* have their roots in the notion of pledge, in the sense of vowing a solemn oath and of one who becomes a hostage or bail for another. This history resonates with Levinas's notion of ethical subjectivity as pledge or hostage.

It is also significant that Kant's word for duty, *Pflicht*, originally referred to social or community bonds forged through care and dependency. *Pflicht* comes from *Pflëgen*, which means care for or look after and has strong connotations of community.[2] There is, then, care, dependency, community, and social bondage, so to speak, already contained within Kant's notion of duty as *Pflicht* or plight. Thinking of Kant's *Pflicht* as plight sets us on a path that leads more directly to Levinas. More important, however, it gives us a different way to reconcile ethics and politics. For *plight* means "bind," not only in the sense of pledge, as in vowing an oath, but also in the sense of intertwining, plaiting, or braiding. Ethics and politics are bound in this sense of intertwining, both conceptually and practically. Indeed, we might even say that their necessary relationship puts us in a double bind, and this is the post-Kantian plight of ethics.

In the history of moral philosophy culminating in our moment of hyperbolic ethics, our plight has become less familiar and more uncanny, as the notion of duty or obligation increasingly takes on the sense of risk and urgency involved in substituting myself for another in a way that entails danger, even becoming a hostage. *Hostage* also has its roots in a Latin word for pledge—*pledge* in the sense of giving oneself over for the other, and also in the sense of making a promise or a binding oath; a speech act, the very possibility of which assumes both other people and the Other of language and culture. Kant's autonomous will gives way to the vulnerability of the face, for Levinas, or suffering as the uncanny "capacity" for vulnerability, for Derrida. The "I can" of moral agency becomes passively subjected to the other upon whom it depends ontologically and biologically for its very existence. Levinas proposes a responsibility that I cannot refuse because there is no *I* without it. Insofar as I am, I am answerable and responsible to and for the other. *Contra* Hegel and Sartre, Levinas (1998) maintains that subjectivity is not the in-itself become for-itself but, rather, the in-itself become for-the-other. Yet Levinas insists that this hyper-ethical responsibility operates on a level opposed to the political. Justice, he says, requires a third, whereas the force of our ethical obligation finds its imperative in the face-to-face relation, which cannot be translated into the political realm.

If Kant reconciles ethics and politics by appealing to the rationality and goodness of God, for Levinas ethics and politics couldn't be further apart, precisely because of the relationship between the ethical face-to-face and God as infinite. Ethics is of the singular, unique, infinite, and untranslatable, an encounter with absolute alterity, whereas justice or politics is generalizable, finite, necessarily translatable, and requires arbitrators of civil codes. For Levinas, the gap between ethics and politics could not be wider (Levinas 1989). So how do we get from the Kantian concept of duty with its source in reason to the Levinasian notion of responsibility as "the essential, primary and fundamental structure of subjectivity" (1985, 95)? In our attempt to untangle, and thereby rebind, ethics and politics, in order to forge the untranslatable singularity of each to the necessity of generalizable civil codes, it is significant that the word *responsibility* itself was first used in relation to politics and not to ethics. Specifically, in both English and French, the word has its origins in late-eighteenth-century discussions of government and civil law. The *Oxford English Dictionary* locates the first use of *responsibility* in debates on the U.S. Constitution in the Federalist Papers of 1787. And the first use of the French *responsabilité*—the very word repeatedly used by Levinas and Derrida—appears around the same time and refers to the responsibility of government and government officials.[3] Just as we have found care, community, and dependency on others contained within the history of Kant's concept of duty, we find political and juridical law contained within the history of Levinas's concept of responsibility and his ethics as first philosophy.

When the concept of responsibility moves into philosophy proper in the nineteenth century, it is not as an ethical concept but, rather, as a political one, which again refers to principles of law and government, specifically punishment, or what John Stuart Mill calls "punishability" and what F. H. Bradley calls "accountability" (see McKeon 1957, 6–7). Paul Ricoeur traces this slippage in the juridical concept of responsibility from responsibility as *attribution* to responsibility as *retribution* through the term *account*, which links imputation to responsibility. Specifically, Ricoeur cites a 1771 legal dictionary: "To impute an action to someone is to attribute it to him as its actual author, to put it, so to speak, on his account and to make him responsible for it" (2000, 14). In Ricoeur's terms, responsibility as accountability suggests "the idea of a kind of *moral bookkeeping* of merits and demerits, as in a double-entry ledger: receipts and expenses, credits and debits," wherein "the metaphor of a balance book seems to underlie the apparently banal idea of being accountable for, and the . . . idea of giving an account, in the sense of reporting, recounting" (Ricoeur 2000, 14; my emphasis). In other words, in its juridical origins, responsibility is a matter of calculation and accounting on the scales of justice, such that punishments are compensations or payments for crimes committed. Ricoeur points out that responsibility owes its associations with payment to a theological context, Saint Paul's interpretation of the crucifixion of Christ as payment for original sin.

The Death Penalty as Kantian Duty or Regulative Ideal?

It is perhaps no coincidence, then, that the word *responsibility* first appears in these juridical writings at the very same time that Kant produces his most powerful articulations of the metaphysics of morals, in which he reconciles morals and politics through a kind of strict "moral bookkeeping" based on the principle of equality contained in the notion of *lex talionis*, or justice as retribution. Although lex talionis also takes us back to the Judeo-Christian doctrine of an eye for an eye and a tooth for a tooth found in the Old Testament (and ultimately Kant, too, grounds its absolute authority on the benevolence of a rational God), Kant is clear that the retaliation required by the law of talionis cannot be based on revenge; but, rather, it must be based on equality. The word that Kant uses for equality is *Gleichheit*, which also connotes *likeness*. To be fair, the punishment must fit the crime in the sense of *like for like*. In both his moral theory and his political theory, Kant insists on the connection between freedom and equality. Moreover, as we know, he maintains that morality requires that we do our duty for its own sake and not from inclinations or emotions alone. Kant explicitly opposes to the mechanisms of nature the freedom that he claims confers dignity on humans. In spite of this, Nietzsche criticizes Kant's "economic justification of virtue," which makes morality a matter of mechanically following laws (Nietzsche 2003, 176; cf., e.g., Kant 1996a, 340–41).

Arguably, however, the strictness of Kant's concepts of duty and equality is related to his insistence that lex talionis or retribution must be devoid of vengeance. Moral bookkeeping and mechanical principles are ways of trying to ensure an equality that does not allow us to unjustly favor those we love and torture those we hate. In this way, we could say that in spite of his various appeals to God, Kant attempts to salvage lex talionis from its vengeful Judeo-Christian roots. For Kant, the ultimate test for the strict principle of talionis, or like for like, is the death penalty. Interestingly, rather than interpret the death penalty as exchanging one life for another— life for life—Kant sees *giving death* as the necessary demand of the principle of talionis: "There is no *similarity* between life, however wretched it may be, and death, hence no likeness between the crime and the retribution unless death is judicially carried out upon the wrongdoer." So a life of hard labor or in prison is never like death. Thus Kant concludes that if an offender "has committed murder he must *die*." And, furthermore, he maintains that "the best equalizer before public justice is *death*" (1996, 474–75; emphasis in original). A death for a death is demanded by the principle of equality, which is the ground not only for both moral and civil law but also for Kant's first article of perpetual peace. The very concept of moral law that binds politics to ethics, then, is based on the principle of equality as like for like, which ultimately depends upon the death penalty, a death for a death, and the state's sovereign right to put to death.

With Kant, we have what Derrida recognizes as the most *philosophical* argument for the death penalty. Kant's is a principled argument, and Derrida demands a principled response. Kant's analysis is based on concepts of duty, dignity, and sovereignty, the very concepts that Derrida uses to undermine Kant's conclusions. Furthermore, following those Kantian principles to their logical conclusions—or, we could say, taking up those concepts in their pure forms—Derrida's analysis suggests that even for Kant, the death penalty may be a regulative ideal that we cannot and should not ever achieve. Derrida argues that the role of the death penalty in Kant's philosophy is paradoxical insofar as it both founds all criminal law and punishment, and is itself a form of punishment. One result is that the death penalty becomes a sort of transcendental absolute required for all law and state sovereignty: "There would be no more law, and above all no criminal law, without the mechanism of the death penalty, which is thus its condition of possibility, its transcendental, if you like (at once internal, included: the death penalty is an element of criminal law, one punishment among others, a bit more severe to be sure; and external, excluded: a foundation, a condition of possibility, an origin, a non-serial exemplarity, hyperbolic, more and other than a penalty). It is this transcendentalization that a consistent abolitionism must take on" (Derrida 2004, 142). In Derrida's view, Kant's argument is circular: Kant both argues for the death penalty as a form of punishment based on the logic of lex talionis and views the death penalty as the ultimate foundation of that logic.

Moreover, Derrida asks what kind of penalty is death. He seems to ask, How can death, a supposed natural event (or nonevent), be a punishment? Discussing the ambiguities of the French word for penalty, *peine*, Derrida argues that (in French at least) it is not so easy to distinguish between *peine* as punishment or penalty and *peine* as pain or even revenge, precisely what the Kantian argument for the death penalty as the great equalizer attempts to avoid (see Dutoit 2012). As Thomas Dutoit puts it in his analysis of Derrida's 1999–2001 seminar on the death penalty, "because the word *peine* can mean the penalty, the punishment, as well as the pain, it can be difficult to hold them separate from each other when one is variously discussing the distinction, say, between a legal punishment (*poena forensis*) and what, because it is merely natural, is an act of revenge, as in the *poena naturalis* (when a group of people lynch someone rather than allow the courts to determine what is to be done)" (Dutoit 2012).

Dutoit offers the following translation of a paragraph from one of the seminar lectures, in which Derrida challenges our certainty about "death" and "penalty," let alone "death penalty":

> What is it, this thing, the death penalty [*la peine de mort*]? Is it a penalty, a punishment [*une peine*]? ... And what if the death penalty [*la peine de mort*] were an untenable artifact, a pseudo-concept, such that the two terms, penalty [*peine*] and death, punishment [*peine*] and capital, did not let themselves be joined, like an out of joint syntagm, and such that it would be necessary to choose between the penalty and death without one being able ever to justify their logical grammar, except by unjustifiable violence, so much so that it would be necessary to choose between the penalty and death? (Lecture 13, December 13, 2000, typescript pp. 2–3; quoted in Dutoit 2012)

Dutoit comments, "Derrida brings out that to put 'penalty' (punishment, pain) and 'death' together is a monstrous hybrid. Either one chooses 'penalty,' in which case one lets go of death: the convict does not get put to death; or one chooses death, which is not a punishment, a pain or a penalty, since all of those presuppose life, continued life. The 'death penalty' is impossible, an impossible concept, the existence of which and the legal theory of which, are both based on an 'unjustifiable violence,' a forcing together of law and nature as if this were possible" (Dutoit 2012).

In *For What Tomorrow* Derrida describes and deconstructs the Kantian distinction between *poena naturalis* and *poena forensic*: "The founding distinction of the concept of 'punishment' in Kant, i.e., the difference between (a) *poena naturalis*, a punishment, entirely interior and private, which the guilty party can inflict on himself, before all law and institutions, and (b) *poena forensis*, punishment strictly speaking, administered from the outside by society, through its judicial apparatus and its historical institutions" (Derrida 2004, 150). This distinction between penalty as social or cultural and pain as private or natural (along with the various meanings or types of penalties and pains) is just one of the places where Derrida puts pressure on what is essential to the Kantian argument. Another such pressure point is the related distinction between punishment by the state, or hetero-punishment, and self-punishment, or auto-punishment; in other words, what comes down to the distinction between execution and suicide.

Following the logic of Kant's argument, someone who is guilty, by definition, must recognize his guilt and therefore *will* his own punishment;

in the case of murder, he must will the death penalty. Derrida argues, "The distinction between self-punishment and hetero-punishment: the guilty party, as a person and a rational subject, should, according to Kant, understand, approve, even call for the punishment—including the supreme penalty; this transforms all institutional and rational punishment coming from outside (*forensis*) into automatic and autonomous punishment or into the indiscernible confines of interior punishment (*poena naturalis*). . . . But here one can no longer distinguish, in all rigor, the sphere of pure immune law, intact, not contaminable by everything we would want to purify it of: interest, passion, vengeance, revenge, the sacrificial drive" (Derrida 2004, 150). Derrida is clear: he is not saying that for Kant execution is the same as suicide, but rather that the distinction cannot be maintained within Kant's own logic. Moreover, the very elements that Kant insists must be excluded from arguments for (and the practice of) capital punishment come back with a vengeance, so to speak.

Another place where Derrida puts pressure on Kant's argument is in terms of the exceptions that Kant grants to the supposedly categorical demand for a death for a death, including a mother killing her infant. These exceptions point to the limitations of the logic of lex talionis or the law of retribution as an "eye for an eye." Derrida argues, "Kant fails, in my view, on questions that are moreover often sexual, on sex crimes—pederasty, rape, bestiality—to produce a principle of equivalence, and therefore of calculability" (Derrida 2004, 151). For these crimes, Kant's adherence to lex talionis makes it difficult for him to set out punishments equal to the crimes. He does not want to say that the rapist should be raped or that the perpetrator of infanticide should be herself killed. Derrida challenges the very possibility of lex talionis as a calculation of equivalencies when he says, "the question of the death penalty is not only that of the political onto-theology of sovereignty; it is also, around this calculation of an impossible equivalence between crime and punishment, their incommensurability, an impossible evaluation of debt" (151). It becomes a question of accounting, and when it does so, as we have seen, it ceases to be ethical. Indeed, all of the tensions between ethics and politics take us back to the incommensurability between the incalculable and the calculable, the asymmetrical and the equivalent.

Kant cannot universalize the principle of the death penalty and at the same time allow for exceptions. One particular exception central to his argument, and to the conceptual problems with capital punishment and the state's sovereignty over life and death, is the exception Kant makes for the sovereign himself. As we have seen, for Kant the sovereignty of the state depends upon the sovereignty of the head of state, which means that the head of state cannot be subjected to its laws. In other words, since he *is* the law, he is above the law. Kant argues that it is better to assassinate the head of state than bring him to trial and execute him. For Kant, trying the sovereign is a challenge to the sovereignty of the state itself. Derrida comments, "Kant gives the example of Charles I and Louis XVI, and goes so far as to judge assassination without trail or abdication of the king less unjustifiable [than formal execution]. That is what is changing in this regard today: the new possibility of judging a head of state, a former head of state, or of summoning him before an international tribunal; to a certain extent, which is in any case very complicated, this calls back to the question the very principle of sovereignty" (2004, 89). Furthermore, he asks, "[D]id the king die?" (90). For if by definition the king is above the law insofar as he is sovereign, and if, as Kant insists, the execution of the king is in principle impossible, then the body of a man was killed, but was it the king? This conceptual issue gets to the heart of political sovereignty. And again it points to the tension between moral and political sovereignty that continues to plague Kant.

Given recent events, including the assassination (if we can call it that) of Osama Bin Laden, the Kantian distinction between execution and assassination is apt. Who can be executed today is telling. Most executions take place in the United States and the Middle East. In the United States, black men are executed at a higher rate than are white men. It is also interesting, as Derrida suggests, that there is a coincidence in Europe between the abolition of the death penalty and international law holding heads of state accountable for crimes, in other words, putting them within reach of the law: "There is doubtless nothing fortuitous in the fact that at the very moment when the immunity of heads of states or armies is being, let us say to remain prudent, called into question by international criminal authorities, we know that, whatever the worst crimes they are accused of, the accused will never again be condemned to death" (2004, 152).

While Derrida mentions various empirical facts, such as this one, he is primarily concerned with a *principled* argument against the death penalty. He spends so much time with Kant because Kant attempts to provide a principled argument for the death penalty (cf. Dutoit 2012). Derrida maintains, "As long as the flaws of such a line of argument are not made to appear from the inside, in the rigor of concepts; as long as a discourse of the Kantian or Hegelian type, which claims to justify the death penalty in a principled way, without concern for interest, without reference to the least utility, is not 'deconstructed,' we will be confined to a precarious, limited abolitionist discourse, conditioned by empirical facts and, in its essence, provisional in relation to a particular context, situated within a logic of means and ends, falling short of strict juridical rationality" (2004, 150). As we will see, this is precisely what is at stake in the protests against the execution of Troy Davis and the celebrations of the execution of Lawrence Brewer. Although the unjust practice and unjust application of the death penalty can and should be powerful challenges to it, in order to abolish it *as such* we need a principled argument. In other words, although racism, the conviction and execution of innocent men, and the failure of technologies to ensure that the condemned do not suffer are crucial arguments for abolitionists, we also need a principled argument against the death penalty in and of itself, because otherwise its justification appears to be merely a matter of fixing a broken system, or of properly applying a sound principle.

Returning to Kant's principled argument for the death penalty, Derrida continues to challenge it by exposing its theological roots, which makes the argument not a properly philosophical one but rather a religious one. Derrida claims, "Kant's reinterpretation of the lex talionis" powerfully reactivates biblical and Roman traditions by displacing them (2004, 151). He argues that both the death penalty and philosophies of sovereignty are ultimately grounded in theological principles based on a transcendent God, an eternal soul, and an afterlife. As we have seen, Derrida reminds us that the universal commandment "Thou shalt not kill" is at odds with the equally universal commandment "An eye for an eye," or lex talionis, that demands the death penalty in the name of God (see Derrida 2002a, 86, and 2004, 140). In more practical terms, Derrida points out, "almost everywhere, as statistics show, those who are the most violently opposed to voluntary termination of pregnancy, those who sometimes try to kill doctors in the name of the 'right' to life, those very people are often the most ardent supporters of the death penalty. . . . These so-called unconditional defenders of life are just as often militants for death" (2004, 140).

We have a toxic combination of conceptual reliance on theological principles that require the death penalty and religious fundamentalism that kills in the name of life. Derrida reminds us that Socrates, Christ, Joan of Arc, and Al-Hallaj were all executed on the basis of a religious accusation in the name of some sacred law; the state then took up the charge founded in religious authority and condemned and punished the accused (see 2004, 144). In this way, the state also shores up its authority through appeals to the ultimate authority, God. Legally—and the very possibility of law depends on it—the right to take a life, whether in war or by the death penalty, can only be sanctioned in principle (as opposed to in practice) by appeals (implicitly or explicitly) to the authority of God (cf. Derrida 2004, 88). Moreover, the transfer of His absolute authority to his "representatives" on earth is necessary to justify taking someone's life in war or as a punishment. Otherwise, these "enemies" or "criminals" must be left to God's judgment, which mere mortals cannot know or anticipate.

As we have seen, Derrida argues that the death penalty and sovereignty are built on the same scaffolding. Thus, any deconstruction of one must necessarily be a deconstruction of the other (2004, 88). Indeed, Derrida makes the much more radical claim that the death penalty is the keystone of speculative philosophy. Recall this passage from *For What Tomorrow*:

> For a long time I have thus been persuaded that the deconstruction of the speculative scaffolding (not to mention the scaffold) that upholds the philosophical discourse on the death penalty is not one necessity among others, a particular point of application. If one could speak here of an architectonic and of edification, the death penalty would be the keystone or, if you prefer, the cement, the weld, as I just said, of the onto-theological-political, the prosthetic artifact that keeps its upright, along with the nature-technique distinction and everything that follows from it (*physis/tekhne, physis/nomos, physis/thesis*), a non-natural thing, a historical law, a properly and strictly human and supposedly rational law. (2004, 148)

Apart from revenge or deterrence, the death penalty is consistent with, if not justified by, the traditional philosophical and religious separation between body and soul. For some, the death penalty is seen to purify the soul. Kant, for example, insists that the criminal as a rational agent should not only acknowledge his crimes and accept his punishment, but should also will it for himself (his own rational sovereignty depends upon his willing it for himself) (150). The death of the earthly body is necessary for the sake of the eternal soul or faculty of reason itself. On this view, this is why animals cannot be subject to the death penalty—because they do not have reason or souls. In addition, the scaffolding of the death penalty is the support for sovereignty in the sense that the king or the sovereign has the power to put to death, or to let die. Derrida argues that for Kant all law comes back to this principle; namely, that the sovereign must have the power to kill. And, as Derrida points out, even after the death penalty has been abolished in Europe, the police continue to kill suspects without trial and soldiers continue to kill enemies in war. Although he insists that we not confuse these different types of killing, the point is that the sovereign government maintains the right to kill even without the death penalty.

Hyperbolic Ethics and *Deconstructive Politics*

While Derrida deconstructs Kant's argument for the death penalty, in a certain sense he embraces Kant's cosmopolitan ideal of hospitality. Indeed he uses this ideal against justifications of state violence, including capital punishment. Claiming to be "more Kantian than Kant," Derrida says that there is no concept of hospitality without the notion of pure hospitality, even if all instances of that concept are corrupted (e.g., 2004, 60).[4] Yet he also criticizes Kant's conditions of universal hospitality insofar as they are tied to the nation-state and because they are conditional. He says, "[T]his concept of cosmopolitan hospitality, as respectable and always perfectible as it is, seems to me to be still bound to a figure of citizenship in the nation-state, the very one that now finds itself in a process of dislocation, transgression, transformation" (2004, 97). Derrida goes further: "When I speak of democracy to come—this thing that can appear a little mad or impossible—I am thinking of a democracy that would no longer be bound in any essential way to citizenship" (97). Democracy beyond citizenship. Hospitality beyond nation-states. Derrida evokes a democracy and hospitality to come, not just as regulative ideals, but also and moreover as urgent pleas for a more ethical politics, beyond the sovereignty of the state with its inherent right over the life and death of both its own citizens and its enemies.

Derrida counterposes what he calls "unconditional hospitality" to the conditioned forms of hospitality of Kant and of everyday life. He maintains that pure unconditional forgiveness or pure unconditional hospitality—those that are "worthy of their names"—are always contaminated with auto-affection, concern for self, and projections onto others. Yet this distinction between self and other becomes one of the most profound oppositions subjected to Derrida's deconstruction, or to deconstructive ethics. And it is precisely this deconstruction of the self-other dichotomy that puts pressure on the seeming opposition between ethics and politics, whether ethics obligation originates in the self (à la Kant) or in the other (à la Levinas).

Discussing the tense, but necessary, relationship between unconditional and conditioned hospitality, Derrida says, "[I]t is the pure and hyperbolical hospitality in whose name we must always invent the best dispositions, the least bad conditions. . . . Calculate the risks, yes, but don't shut the door on what cannot be calculated, meaning the future of the foreigner" (2005, 67). Politics necessitates calculation, perhaps even cost-benefit or risk analysis, while ethics needs universal principles. Ethics demands the unconditional, while politics always requires conditions. Perhaps in order to "avoid the worst," as Derrida sometimes says, we need to embrace what remains a secret, what cannot be calculated or even anticipated and thereby prevents us from ever thinking, or understanding, or knowing once and for all the meanings of hospitality, justice, or democracy. To think the secret is to think the impossibility of knowing, the impossibility of articulating, and perhaps even the impossibility of ethics itself. And yet this attempt to think the impossible, to articulate the impossible, may be the very condition of possibility for ethics, insofar as it must operate within the world of real politics and yet cannot be reduced to that world. Derrida's notions of justice and democracy to come try to maintain the tense but necessary relation between ethics and politics, for the sake of a more ethical politics.

THE DECONSTRUCTIVE DOSE

The deconstructive machine is one that necessarily turns back on itself. Or, more precisely, it is the operation of turning the machinery of liberal democracy and Western intellectual history back on themselves. Deconstructive ethics operates according to the logic of "one nail takes out the other"; it is a machine with which to challenge and surprise the other machination, the machination of violence. As I have argued elsewhere, this deconstructive turning back is a homeopathic operation (see Oliver 2007). For example, take the concept of purity itself. In *Of Grammatology*,

Derrida probes the limit set up between various binary oppositions, including nature and culture, in order to challenge the "mythic purity" of concepts (good or evil) on either side of the divide: "Man calls himself man only by drawing limits excluding his other from the play of supplementarity: the *purity* of nature, of animality, primitivism, childhood, madness, divinity. The approach to these limits is at once feared as a threat of death, and desired as access to a life without differance" (1976, 244, my emphasis; cf. 1976, 235, 290). Derrida's deconstructive project challenges our investment in the purity of concepts that drive the history of philosophy. Yet in his later work on forgiveness and hospitality, Derrida insists on the purity of these concepts. In order to explain this apparent shift, we could say that Derrida employs a concept of purity *homeopathically* in these later writings. The concept of *purity*—or we could say the purity of concepts—that he employs in his later work seems intended to counteract the history of philosophy's adherence to a notion of pure nature as distinct from impure or corrupt culture.

For example, in "On Forgiveness," Derrida uses a notion of pure forgiveness to interrupt discourses of racial and ethnic purity as manifested in the Holocaust and apartheid (cf. Oliver 2007). On the one hand, Derrida challenges the possibility of forgiveness as it operates in contemporary discussions of "crimes against humanity." On the other, he "measures" such crimes against the immeasurable, or as he says, incalculable, concept of pure forgiveness. He suggests that only by comparing our everyday forms of forgiveness that operate within economies of exchange and reciprocity to the concept of pure forgiveness can we continue to challenge ourselves or open ourselves to the most radically other, whom we may not even recognize, let alone to forgive. Indeed, pure forgiveness is not a matter of one's ability; it is not something that one gives or takes away, at least not if it is forgiveness "worthy of its name," which is to say worthy of the concept of forgiveness itself.

In this way, Derrida's notion of pure forgiveness serves as a *homeopathic* remedy for genocidal discourses of racial and ethnic purity. The homeopathic remedy, if never a cure, requires taking a dose of the very poison we seek to neutralize: we need a dose of one kind of purity—pure or natural purity—as an antidote to another kind of purity: one ideal of purity takes out the other. Unlike the discourses of purity that feed racial cleansing and genocide, Derrida's is a conceptual purity, or better yet, the concept of purity, or the pure concept with which he contrasts all corrupted forms. He is not holding out an impossible ideal so that we may always feel inferior or ashamed, but rather so that we will also be open to reconsidering what we take to be hospitality, forgiveness, democracy, or justice. His deconstructive dose of purity uses reason against itself in this homeopathic way as an antidote to all of the reasons human beings have given to justify enslaving each other and other living creatures. Even from his earliest work, deconstruction has been a homeopathic methodology insofar as it has always used the text, the concepts, and the history of philosophy against itself in order to begin to imagine an ethics "worthy of its name" (cf. Oliver 2007).

Derrida's addition of the phrase "worthy of its name" ("*digne de ce nom*") to his invocations of the pure concepts of forgiveness and hospitality suggests that we consider what is proper to the concept or the name. Here again, however, Derrida uses one economy of property or propriety against another. Pure forgiveness worthy of its name is forgiveness that is proper or fitting to the concept of forgiveness, to the name forgiveness, as it has evolved in Western thought. *Pure* forgiveness *worthy* of its name, then, doubly emphasizes the value of the pure concept or name to which we aspire and for which we must remain vigilant. That is, we can never rest content that we have achieved our goals of hospitality, forgiveness, or justice. This is why Derrida also insists on the *unconditional* (a word that he also repeatedly uses) form of these concepts, if there is such a thing (a phrase he also sometimes uses).

Derrida's discourse of pure concepts interrupts one discourse of property, purity, and rigor with another. He uses the notion of pure concepts as an antidote to any self-satisfied everyday practices of forgiveness, including political practices such as South Africa's Truth and Reconciliation Commission. On the one hand, the pure concepts of hospitality, forgiveness, and justice require unconditionality, and in that they are impossible to put into practice. On the other hand, all instances of hospitality, forgiveness, and justice have meaning only in relation to their pure or unconditional concepts: "Only an unconditional hospitality can give meaning and practical rationality to a concept of hospitality. Unconditional hospitality exceeds juridical, political, or economic calculation. But no thing and no one happens or arrives without it" (Derrida 2005, 149).

As it plays out in Derrida's work, this dynamic of purity and contamination issues from the impossible relationship between the unconditional and the conditioned. How can we inscribe the unconditional or infinite within the conditioned and finite? This is the ethical question par excellence. We must at once acknowledge the impossibility of this task and recognize that all of our attempts are contaminated. Yet, as Derrida repeatedly reminds us, this paradoxical situation exonerates no one. To the contrary, it is the heart of ethical responsibility.[5] The acknowledgment of impossibility or contamination should not lead to quietude or despair. Rather, it should lead to vigilance and to a renewed commitment to hyperbolic ethics, to recognizing that our ethical obligations may be to others whom we do not yet or even cannot recognize.

In a sense, Derrida's deconstructive ethics provides a kind of corrective for morality.[6] Moral imperatives made and followed by the sovereign "I am" or "I can" are at odds with ethics. Moral codes may give us a clear sense of our duties, but they do so by turning response into mindless reactions that avoid the difficulty of ethical decision making, including the existential ambiguity of ethics discussed by Beauvoir, the insomnia of ethical responsibility suggested by Levinas, the ambiguity and ambivalence of Kristeva's notion of abjection as the flip side of morality, and the crucial process of Derridean undecidability out of which decisions emerge. If morality divides the world into good and evil, or natural and perverse (or as we will see, divides it between the *unjustly executed* Troy Davis and the *justly executed* Lawrence Brewer), then hyperbolic ethics demands that we constantly question those binary oppositions and our own investments in them. Do we make such distinctions in order to foster nourishing and healthful relationships, or do we divide the world in order to conquer it and take others as trophies? (cf. Oliver 2007). In terms more familiar to recent discussions in ethics, we might ask: Do we circumscribe differences to justify hierarchies and domination, or to respect differences and acknowledge their value? More Derridean questions are: How can we tell the difference? And who is this *we*, anyhow?

In *On the Name*, Derrida asks, "critique of self, but critique of whom exactly? To whom would the reflexive be returned?" (1995b, 13). If deconstructive ethics is a vigilant self-critique of our own most cherished values and of our limitations, then we also have to apply it to the notions of *our own*, *ours*, *us*, and *we*. For aren't those categories precisely the ones at stake in Derrida's upping the ante? *Us* or *them*, *friend* or *enemy*, *good* or *evil?* . . . How can *we* be so sure *we* can tell the difference? Moreover, who is this *we?* These are some of the most difficult and dizzying questions of slow and differentiated deconstruction. But they are also the questions that raise the stakes of ethical and political life. And, if "we" are willing to take the risk, to subject ourselves to the deconstructive machine, our following of its circuitous and difficult rhythms may "pay off" in unexpected ways.

The Psychoanalytic Supplement

Deconstruction is one way of continually leaving open this "we." But in order to begin to understand why we divide the world into us versus them, and how we do so, I suggest that we must turn to psychoanalysis. Why and how we divide the world into friend or enemy, good or evil, is a question for psychoanalysis. It is a question of avowing our own investments in violence and death penalties of all sorts. To return to where I began this chapter, we could say that psychoanalytic avowal is another form of plight or pledge in the sense of vowing an oath to admit and explore our own economic and psychic investments in the violence we say that we abhor. This is particularly relevant when we feel outraged or wronged and want payback. Recall the "with us or against us" reactions to September 11, 2001, and the continued political discourse on "hunting down" terrorists and "making them pay." Think, too, of all of the revenge fantasies—too many to begin to list—that populate our cultural imaginary as evidenced by popular media, including a new TV soap opera aptly titled *Revenge*.

In addition to indulging in self-righteous indignation and outrage, we need to examine our own economic and psychic investments in, and dependence on, state-sanctioned violence, killing, and war. For example, directly or indirectly, many of us receive our paychecks from the very state governments that are executing people and from the federal government that is sending soldiers off to kill and be killed. As my grandmother used to say, rather than accuse someone else for the stink all around us, "the fox should smell his own hole first." This goes not only for Kant's serpents, those clever politicians, but also and even more so for Kant's doves, those supposedly guileless moralists. After all, Kant's serpents and doves originally found their home in Christ's instructions to his disciples in the New Testament: "Behold, I send you forth as sheep in the midst of wolves: be ye therefore as wise as serpents, and harmless as doves" (King James Bible, Matthew 10:16).

This expanding bestiary, warning us against our fellow man by reminding us of our own animality, is another signal that we need psychoanalysis to begin to understand our fears and desires as social creatures. But when we add the psychoanalytic postulation of unconscious fears and desires, our ethical and political responsibilities become even more complicated and more acute. For we become responsible not only for our actions, or our intentions à la Kant, our beliefs and emotions à la Sartre, and those of the other à la Levinas, but also for our own unconscious fears and desires, which remain hidden even from us.

If Derrida's hyperbolic ethics puts us in a double bind between laws that require equality and radical alterity—we must decide in favor of justice even though pure justice is impossible, even though we cannot know, and even though any decision we make can be corrupt or corrupted—then psychoanalysis may be the only way to navigate between these conflicting obligations; namely, obligations to respect the dignity of each, not only in Kant's sense of universal equality, but also in Levinas's sense of singularity, which takes us beyond equality to asymmetrical responsibility. Psychoanalysis gives us a way of addressing the tension between politics based on law and ethics based on radical alterity. It may help spring the trap of this double bind between ethics and politics by giving us the tools to critically examine how we project our unconscious fears and desires onto others whom we call foreigners, enemies, monsters deserving some form of death penalty. A hyperbolic ethics born from psychoanalysis commands us to investigate how we distribute dignity, equality, and respect such that some profit while others pay the price. The psychoanalytic supplement to hyperbolic ethics binds ethics to politics without appeals to the sovereignty of the will or of God, but rather through the interminable process of analyzing the ways in which we disavow and avow our investments in violence and cruelty.

Without sovereignty and without ownership, we are responsible for what we cannot and do not control, for our unconscious fears and desires and their effects on others. The fragile hope is that by acknowledging the death drive within ourselves, we can begin to prevent killing and never give up trying to find ways to abolish death penalties in all their forms. The death drive is not the Kantian notion of death as the great equalizer, but rather the tension in life itself, both destructive and creative, always con-joined with both pleasure and pain, joy and sorrow, and the ambiguities of life that not only exceed, but also expose, the fantasy of death as an absolute end point, or final resting place. Far from the perpetual peace of the Dutch innkeeper's sign with which Kant ironically opens his "Toward Perpetual Peace: A Philosophical Sketch," the death drive is the force that fuels the fantasy of the end of life as everlasting peace.

Is philosophy, perhaps all philosophy, ultimately founded on the absolute certainty of death, that we are all, in one way or another, sentenced to death? From Socrates becoming a martyr for his philosophical ideals to Heidegger insisting that Dasein is unique in its being-towards-death, philosophy seems preoccupied with death. In *The Beast and the Sovereign* volume 2, and in his death penalty seminars, Derrida demonstrates how philosophy is bound to death and the death penalty. Yet in his last seminar, while powerfully calling into question the meaning of death and who can die, Derrida also appeals to the fact that every living being dies as perhaps the ultimate ethical bind (2011). Has death, then, as the absolute and only equalizer, replaced the absolute authority of God, whether Kant's rational God or Levinas's Other God? The death penalty as executed in this country makes clear that both ethics and politics demand that we think through our own death drive rather than bank on the fantasy of equality through death, the fantasy of instant death, or the fantasy of death as the final and absolute resting place. To do so covers over the differences between deaths and death penalties—to be blunt—between so many ways of dying and so many ways of being executed, assassinated, or killed.

SEVERED HEADS

Speaking of blunt, it is telling that the inventors of the guillotine, Doctors Antoine Louis and Joseph-Ignace Guillotin, claimed that the decapitating blade offered the "principle of equality" for death (cf. Kristeva 2012, 91). Guillotin's invention, which he called his "goddaughter," supposedly pro-vided a cleaner, painless death that he maintained gave "at most, the impres-sion of a fresh breeze on the neck" (Kristeva 2012, 92). The idea of a cleaner death was part of the move towards a more modern death, which today has taken the shape of high-tech death, not only in the theater of death used in U.S. prisons, but also in the theater of war with high-tech surgical strikes.

In *The Severed Head,* Julia Kristeva argues that in the case of the guillotine, "the claims of a painless technique and democratic equality immediately merged with metaphysical speculation. . . . [S]ince only what is high
and celestial is attacked at the head, to bring down that head would mean to
prepare another 'beyond.' . . . [D]ecapitation became an esoteric necessity;
indispensible to the emergence of a new head, a new era" (2012, 92–93).[7]
As we have seen, throughout that work, Kristeva argues that the head is
symbolic of thought and of sovereignty, both of the individual, and of the
state. The head is attacked not only in order to institute a new head—King
Louis XIV's head will be replaced not just by another head of state—but
also by a new form of state sovereignty. Indeed, as we have seen, all state
sovereignty depends on the ability to put to death; it authorizes itself
through the death penalty. This recognition is what led Albert Camus to
claim, "To prohibit putting a man to death would be to proclaim publicly
that the society and the State are not absolute values, to decree that nothing
authorizes them to legislate definitively" (quoted in Kristeva 2012, 101).

In a sense, the guillotine ushers in a new era of sovereign justification for
authority over life and death, one that relies on science and technology. The
guillotine, invented by men of science to provide clean, painless death, puts
science in the service of death. And moreover, it feeds the fantasy of technologically mediated instant death. As Kristeva says, "Under the pretext of
scientific interest, a feverish morbidity spread. The spectacle was witnessed,
the taste of blood enjoyed, but even so scientific questions were posed: does
a severed head continue to live? For how long?" (2012, 96). We legitimize
our thirst for violence using science and technology.

And yet the various nicknames given to the guillotine are in excess of its
scientific standing as a high-tech, "painless" machine, supposedly invented
to revolutionize both killing and politics. For example, Derrida discusses
Victor Hugo's obsession with the color red associated with the guillotine,
which he calls "the bloodswigging old crone," and "the infernal scarlet
machine" (2004, 142). Kristeva diagnoses this as the "verbal excitement"
that "accompanies the maniacal cover-up of horror; semantic farce embel-
lishes the progress of technology" (2012, 95). We see the same verbal
excitement around the electric chair, also touted at its inception as the latest
advance in technology, which had the nicknames "sparky" and "ol' yellow,"
among many others, and death by electrocution was called "riding the
lightning." The wordplay and jokes around technologies of execution

suggest that these technologies are more than scientific advances that sustain fantasies of clean and equal death penalties. They are tokens of what Kristeva calls our maniacal cover-up of the horror of capital punishment that allow us to avoid facing head-on, we might say, state-sanctioned murder.

Yet Kristeva also claims that certain fantasies surrounding the guillotine—and we could extend her analysis to technologies of death more generally—not only expose some of the psychic stakes in our investment in capital punishment but also help us to sublimate the violent urges that give rise to it. For example, she says that "only the Marquis de Sade, fierce enemy of the guillotine that he denounces, finds a rhetoric of excess and irony that, here as elsewhere, unveils the erotic fantasies underlying the machinery, to exhaust them in the sudden beauty of a sentence" (2012, 97). Whatever we think of Kristeva's own fascination with the beauty of abject literature and its sublimatory powers, it seems clear from the guillotine's nicknames—"goddaughter," "blood-swigging old crone," "the hungry lady," "Madame Guillotine"—that the guillotine at least is associated with women and sex.

Although the death penalty has been abolished in France, Kristeva argues that the guillotine still haunts the national consciousness, and "political parties allow themselves dark jokes evoking its ghost, and vendettas on all sides are ready to demand the return of capital punishment" (2012, 101). And in the United States, extremist groups claim that the government is planning to use the guillotine to silence its domestic political enemies. The guillotine, then, still slices through imaginary heads and lives on in our imaginary. Moreover, even as the execution of executions has become closed to the public, and in effect hidden from view, it still shows up in spectacular displays on television and in films, particularly in the form of beheading (cf. Derrida 2004, 159). Even state-sanctioned executions have become the stuff of entertainment, especially the suspenseful moment of waiting by the telephone for the governor's pardon—the telephone acting as a technological supplement to capital execution. All of this is to suggest that technologies of death are infused with fantasies, desires, and fears that must be subjected to psychoanalytic interpretations if we are to begin to understand our own investments in these death-bearing technologies.

Psychoanalysis can help us to understand the ways in which science and technology are used to cover over, even disavow, our violent desires. Kristeva suggests that perhaps sadomasochism is the secret of the unconscious.

And if so, she maintains that it must be discharged in language or art not only in order to give it meaning, but also and moreover to help us avoid acting out our violent fantasies. As long as they remain fantasies rather than actions, there is hope. Discussing the Reign of Terror during the French Revolution, she argues, "In opposition to the imaginary intimacy with death, which transforms melancholy or desire into representation and thought, lies the rational realization of the capital act. Vision and action are polar opposites here, and the revolutionary Terror confronts us with that revolting abjection practiced by humanity under the guise of an egalitarian institution of decapitation" (2012, 91). Through art and analysis, as we have seen, Kristeva proposes that we can discharge our desires for capital punishment.

"I am Troy Davis". . . and His Executioner

What, then, are we to make of the fact that currently the United States is the only country in the so-called developed Western world that continues to execute prisoners?[8] As mentioned in the previous chapter, since 1982, the Supreme Court has upheld the use of a tripartite lethal injection protocol as a "humane" method of execution, thereby avoiding the charge that the death penalty constitutes cruel and unusual punishment and thus violates the Eighteenth Amendment. Recall that the first drug to be administered renders the condemned unconscious, the second paralyzes the muscles, and the third kills by stopping the heart. The rationale for rendering the condemned unconscious before killing him is not only to avoid a painful death but also to preserve the *dignity* of the condemned. The dignity in death demanded by the Court, which as we saw in the last chapter is explicit in Justice Roberts's endorsement of the procedure, takes us back to Kant's insistence that the death penalty is necessary in principle, but must be practiced in a way that preserves the condemned person's dignity.

On the one hand, Justice Roberts (with Kant) *imagines* a motionless, emotionless death with dignity. On the other hand, this fantasy of death with dignity, as opposed to other sorts of deaths, undermines Kant's principle of *talionis* wherein death is the great equalizer. For it also indicates that we are not all equal in death, or, at least, that not all deaths are equal.

Indeed, in practice, it is difficult—if not impossible—by the Court's own standards, to determine what a painless, dignified death would entail. What is dignified about being strapped to a gurney against your will, pleading for your life, dying in a theater with spectators watching through a window, losing the ability to speak or to protest, indeed, losing control of all of your bodily functions? In fact, none of us would know. And who is left to testify to his or her own dignity or loss of it with such a death? The paralyzed, motionless form of dignity approved by the Court indicates again that this so-called dignity is produced for the spectators and not out of respect for the condemned.

Even advanced technologies cannot ensure a pain-free, instant death or guarantee that the victim is unconscious at the time of death. In fact, a study of postmortem examinations on prisoners executed by lethal injection concludes that given blood levels of anesthetic, "prisoners may have been capable of feeling pain in almost 90% of cases and may have actually been conscious when they were put to death in over 40% of cases. . . . 43 of the 49 inmates studied were probably sentient, and 21 may have been 'fully aware'" (Motluk 2005). The study continues, "Because a muscle relaxant was used to paralyze them, however, inmates would have been unable to indicate any pain. Ironically," the report continues, "U.S. veterinarians are advised not to use neuromuscular blocking agents while euthanizing animals precisely so they can recognize when the anesthesia is not working" (Motluk 2005). As we have seen, this is not merely a practical problem but also and moreover a philosophical one, because we cannot be certain, from a phenomenological perspective, what counts as "the time of death" or as "consciousness of death."

As I argued in the last chapter, the current three-drug protocol circumvents the very possibility of establishing whether or not the condemned person is suffering or in pain, whether or not he is conscious at the moment of death, and therefore whether or not the punishment is cruel and unusual as defined by the Court. Furthermore, this fabulous fantasy of painless death disavows the reality that we don't know how to define what constitutes consciousness of death, because first-hand testimony is impossible. As long as Lawrence Brewer, recently executed in Texas, goes out snoring as if in a sound sleep (which he apparently did), at some level we can reassure ourselves that his death was the least cruel, most usual, and perhaps even the most desired—namely, dying in one's sleep.

Recently, death penalty abolitionists have turned to what they say is their most powerful argument against the death penalty, namely, the execution of an innocent man, Troy Davis, in Georgia in September 2011. (Davis was found guilty of killing a police officer while attempting to escape the scene of a robbery.) The argument that the criminal justice system can make mistakes, however, is not an argument against the *principle* of the death penalty. Neither is the argument that lethal injection is cruel and unusual. Rather, these arguments allow that although the practice is flawed, the principle may be sound; if only we improve and perfect the practice, then we authorize the principle. The fantasy of humane, painless, instant death—technologically administered—contributes not only to the idea of perfecting the means of death in order to justify the principle of the death penalty, but also to the fantasy of death itself as an *absolute*—in this case, the absolute end of suffering and pain.

Following this line of thought, we might wonder why, leading up to the execution of Davis on September 21, abolitionists around the world rallied and protested, trying to save his life, while at the same time, on that very Wednesday evening, little attention was paid to another execution, that of Lawrence Brewer, the infamous Texan who tied a black hitchhiker to the back of his truck and dragged him to death. He, too, proclaimed his innocence of the murder of James Byrd Jr. until his dying breath. Reportedly there were celebrations of Brewer's death by people who thought that he got what he deserved for his heinous racist hate crime. The outcry against the execution of Davis at the very same moment as the jubilance over the execution of Brewer could be seen as a strangely perverse symptom of the history of racism trying to *put things right* by rejoicing over one execution while raging over the other. Even after the executions, there were comparisons between Davis's refusing a last meal in order to pray silently with friends and family, and Brewer's ordering several pizzas, cheeseburgers, pounds of BBQ, tacos, and other comfort food and then refusing to eat it, which disgusted some commentators and prison officials, who suggested that Brewer was not only undignified but also ungrateful.

Around the world, protesters held signs and wore buttons saying, "I am Troy Davis." But what does it mean to say "I am Troy Davis"? Does this identification with Davis suggest that like him, I am innocent, or that like me, he is? Or that if the state executes him, it executes me; or that if it doesn't execute me, it shouldn't execute him? What does it mean for these protesters around the world, most of them free from prison, most of them white and middle class, to identify with Davis, a condemned black man, raised in poverty, who spent twenty years, half of his life, on death row waiting to be executed? Doesn't this also, at least implicitly, say that I am the victim of the death penalty rather than the perpetrator? After all, the protesters were not holding signs saying "I am Troy Davis's executioner," which they could have done, given that here, and even in France where the death penalty has been abolished since 1981, polls show that most people still favor it. And no one was holding signs saying, "I am Lawrence Brewer." Even though we continue to live in a racist country—the evidence ranges from racist comments directed at President Obama from elected officials at the highest level, to the staggering statistics that show that by far most of the people in prison and on death row are African American, to continued economic inequities reported recently that put the median income for black households well below that of whites (Pear 2011). The toxic combination of economic and social racism creates another type of lethal injection that, in various ways, is killing some people while benefiting others.

I am lingering on this example because perhaps it can help make clear where ethics and politics intersect and intertwine, to the point of putting us in a *bind*, even a *double bind*, reflected in the following series of questions: Can we say not only "I am Troy Davis" but also "I am Troy Davis's executioner" and "I am also Lawrence Brewer and his executioner"? Can we avow our responsibility for, and complicity with, both their crimes and their executions? And what would it take to avow the differences between our comfortable lives and that of Troy Davis? Or, more to the point, to avow that at some level, the comfort of our lives is still dependent upon state-sanctioned killing, including the death penalty in all of its forms, most especially in the forms of institutionalized poverty and state-sanctioned war? What would it take to avow that we are, in some way, also those whom we abhor and those whose actions we disassociate ourselves from in the most adamant ways? That we are, so to speak, our own worst enemies? What would it take to avow that who or whatever they are, our enemies— whether racists like Brewer or terrorists like bin Laden—are also always projections of our own fears and desires? And that whatever they have done, and whatever retaliation we seek, through our fears and desires, often unacknowledged, perhaps even unknown to us, we rationalize our own injustice and justify their torture and death? What would it take to avow that we are part of the ultimate binary killing machine: us versus them, good versus evil, Troy Davis versus Lawrence Brewer?

Public reaction to the executions of Davis and Brewer can and should be analyzed using critical race theory, economics, and social justice theory, along with examining the ethics and politics of capital punishment. But in order to analyze our own investments in death penalties, particularly when we argue against them, even protest against them, we need a psychoanalytic supplement. To understand the effects of killing machines on both the victims and the perpetrators, we need a psychoanalytic supplement to deconstructive hyperbolic ethics. Psychoanalysis may help us to work through the double bind of ethics and politics. Although examining the ways in which economic and political power depend on death penalties is crucial to understanding how they are instituted and why, understanding the ideals and fears behind them is also necessary to put a stop to them. This is why it is important to scrutinize revenge fantasies, especially those that self-righteously proclaim themselves on the side of justice (as in the case of Brewer). To this end, we need to consider the psyche as between reason and unreason, between plight as Kantian duty and responsibility as Levinasian hostage, in order to bind and rebind ethics and politics, by virtue of our sociality that makes us subjects capable of both love and hate, desire and fear. Once we add the postulations of the unconscious to critical philosophy, it becomes necessary to analyze and avow our own psychic investments in state-sanctioned violence, killing, and war.

If, as Kristeva claims, the uncanny strangeness of the unconscious is not only sadomasochistic, but also the "ultimate condition of our being with others" (1991, 192), this haunting togetherness is based neither on Kantian equality as like for like, nor on Levinasian unrecognizable radical alterity. Rather, unconscious fears and desires produce others whom we recognize as friend or enemy, loved or hated, human or animal, virtuous or monstrous, having the right to live or deserving to be put to death. While intimately related to the hyperbolic and impossible ethical demand to open ourselves to the unrecognizable, these categorical oppositions are not simply a matter of our inability to recognize others, or even the otherness of others. Rather, they are a matter of recognizing them as abject others deserving to be locked up, tortured, and killed. We cannot begin to witness to what is beyond recognition in the singularity of each life until we come to terms with the death drive in ourselves, specifically as it manifests itself in our own fears and desires through which we create both our friends and our enemies, both those who are like us and those who are not, both those who are with us, and those who are against us.

Joining hyperbolic ethics with psychoanalysis, then, we might begin to forge ethics and politics in a necessary but tense relation, as the place where we find ourselves: this is our plight as social creatures living together with others. Navigating between Kant's too-easy unification of ethics and politics through universal moral law based on duty, on the one hand, and Levinas's radical separation of the two based on the singularity of infinite ethical responsibility, on the other, let's say that social subjectivity is the thin membrane stretched between infinite ethical responsibility and finite political action. And its depth is the thickness of the flesh in embodied relations with others. Subjectivity is response to others and the environment that binds us to them; and agency is response to social-historical situations, or subject positions, that bind us to the language and culture into which we are born—for better or worse (see Oliver 2001and 2004). Subjective agency is forged through this pledge or bond between politics and ethics made possible, even necessary, by our sociality; we are social embodied animals with fears and desires beyond our control, fears and desires that make love possible, but also make hatred and cruelty realities that we cannot ignore. Our social subjectivity is that thin membrane and that thick embodied relationship with those around us, whether they are animal, vegetable, or mineral, human, beast, or machine . . . or more to the point here, whether they are friend or enemy, loved or hated, welcoming or threatening.

We live in the ethical-political bind between Kantian universality and Levinasian singularity where, without yet having learned the lessons of either, we all-too-easily identify *us* with right and good, and *them* with wrong and evil. This applies just as much to those of us who, from our comfortable living rooms and privileged academic positions, identify with the victims and the oppressed, with Troy Davis, as it does for those who wave flags of victory over the corpses of their enemies, or order the execution of another poor black man sentenced to death. The plight of ethics, then, is not simply figuring out how to relearn our primary-school lesson to share with others in the reciprocity of equality as like for like—no small feat in itself—but also trying to figure out what it would mean to risk sharing the planet with those with whom we do not even share a world. Can we risk avowing our own investments in the very things we so solemnly and self-righteously protest against? Not in order to stop protesting in the name of justice, but rather in the hopes of turning the killing machine back against itself and taking another step toward abolishing death penalties where ever they may be, especially when we find them within ourselves?

INTRODUCTION: MORAL MACHINES AND POLITICAL ANIMALS

1. For general discussions of Derrida and technology and discussions of particular technologies in Derrida, see Clough 2000, Lafontaine 2007, Naas 2010 (he discusses photography), and Prenowtiz 2008 (he discusses the telephone).

2. Indeed, in his later work, Derrida talks about the proximity of Christian fundamentalism's abhorrence of abortion and insistence on capital punishment. This contradiction between advocating life at all costs in one instance, and death at all costs in another, and the invocation of God to justify both, brings together what Derrida describes as the operations of miracle and machine in what too often becomes a deadly embrace (see "Faith and Knowledge," Derrida 2002a; see also Naas 2012).

Like a machine, and now relying on various machines or technologies, religion churns out moral slogans to justify everything from bombing abortion clinics or the World Trade Center, to occupying entire countries through military dominance—all justified through appeals to God. Can the deconstruction machine take on the religion machine? And what would it mean to turn a deconstructive strategy onto religion through new technologies of life and death that also employ science to justify the so-called moral high ground? In "Faith and Knowledge," Derrida argues that science and religion are driven by the same machine, namely, revelation. Religion asks us to accept what we do not see on the faith that it will someday be revealed. Science asks us to accept what we do not see on the knowledge that even now it is being revealed to us. Whether we choose to look through the microscope of science or the lace-veil of religion, we cannot avoid either technology or God, even if they take different forms.

3. There are several works that discuss the machine in Derrida and/or use Derrida's concept of the machine, including Naas 2009 and 2012, Barker 1999, Bass 2006, Critchley 1999, De Ville 2009, Johnson 2008, Lucy 2001, Luke 2003,

Standish 2000, Pettman 2010, and Stiegler 2001. Stiegler traces the machine from Derrida's very earliest work in his Master's thesis on Husserl. In *Miracle and Machine* (2012), Michael Naas gives a beautifully sustained interpretation of Derrida's "Faith and Knowledge," in which he argues that the machine and the miracle are the two sources of religion and science. Bradley 2011 is another important recent contribution to the discussion of the machine in Derrida.

4. For discussions of sovereignty in Derrida's work, see Balke 2005, Cain 2011, Cheah 2009, Mendoza 2011, Goodrich 2008, Gratton 2009, Haddad 2008, Lawlor 2007, Legrande 2009, Leitch 2007, Miller 2008, Naas 2008, 2005, and 2006, Wadiwel 2010, Weber 2008, Williams 2005, and Wood 2008, among others.

5. Indeed, in some ways, it is the difference between those various animals running through and away from his texts and the different machines also running there that preoccupies him. Animals run, and so do machines. And in his first posthumously published work, Derrida turns his deconstructive machine back on the question: Are animals machines? Derrida, the philosophical animal par excellence, uses the resources of his deconstructive project to jam what Giorgio Agamben calls the "anthropological machine" in various ways, including setting the animals free from philosophical confines, that is, from the ways in which philosophers have traditionally described them as being like machines, making humans, and men in particular, grist for that very same mill that has churned out the absolute, fixed, and universal division between man and animal. One way he does so is by introducing the machine on both sides of the man-animal or culture-nature divide, in the hopes of challenging or surprising that other machination (that of the anthropological machine) with the machinations of deconstruction (cf. Agamben 2004).

6. For a discussion of slow and differentiated deconstruction, see Kelly Oliver, "The *Slow and Differentiated* Machinations of Deconstructive Ethics," in Len Lawlor, ed., *Blackwell Companion to Derrida* (Oxford: Blackwell Publishers, 2013).

7. From his early work, Derrida was concerned to challenge the opposition between nature and culture. When applied to political philosophy, the deconstruction of the nature-culture opposition also presents a challenge to philosophies that ground civil law in natural law. Derrida maintains that there is always already a supplement where we take the origin to be. In other words, the reproduction, or technology (the supplement) produces the origin, or nature. As we will see, this becomes clear in Derrida's engagement with Rousseau's discussion of the importance of the role of the mother or mother earth as natural origin, even when Rousseau repeatedly uses surrogate or substitute mothers to make his point.

1. GENETIC ENGINEERING: DECONSTRUCTING *GROWN* VERSUS *MADE*

1. For a discussion of how cloning might affect our notions of the human using Habermas and Derrida, see Egorova and Edgar 2006. See also Mendieta 2003 for a discussion of Habermas and Derrida on cloning.

2. Judith Butler comments on this paradoxical statement: "It would seem that if she can decide, then her gender is, to some extent, a matter of decision. But if she 'is' a woman, then it would seem not to be a decision. The statement contains two different standards for what we think about sex-determination, and it also belies a certain confusion between sex-determination and gender identity. . . . And yet, if we consider that this act of 'sex determination' was supposed to be collaboratively arrived at by a panel that included 'a gynecologist, an endocrinologist, a psychologist and an expert on gender' (why wasn't I called!?), then the assumption is that cultural and psychological factors are part of sex-determination, and that no one of these 'experts' could come up with a definitive finding on his or her own (presuming that binary gender holds). This co-operative venture suggests as well that sex-determination is decided by consensus and, conversely, where there is no consensus, there is no determination of sex. Is this not a presumption that sex is a social negotiation of some kind? And are we, in fact, witnessing in this case a massive effort to socially negotiate the sex of Semenya, with the media included as a party to the deliberations?" (Butler 2009).

3. Even Iris Young, whose essay "Pregnant Embodiment" (2005) has become foundational in feminist interpretations of pregnancy, assumes a freely chosen pregnancy as her starting point, and never considers the phenomenological or existential crisis that getting to that point may require for many women (cf. Lundquist 2008).

4. For a discussion of Derrida and eugenics, see Koshy 2004.

5. As I have argued elsewhere, even a cursory glance through the increasing volume of philosophical literature written on genetic enhancement and grounded in discussions of reproductive choice—authored primarily by prominent mainstream analytic philosophers (who—gender-testing aside—appear to be almost exclusively male)—will shock feminist readers, given the lack of any mention of feminism, the women's movement's decades-long struggles for reproductive choice, or women's subjective experiences of reproduction and reproductive choice. For example, the following book-length studies of reproductive choice based on genetics, including gene therapies, enhancements, and selection, never once mention feminism or acknowledge any inherent relation between their discussions of reproductive choice and the pro-choice movement, even when they mention abortion: Jonathan Glover, *Choosing Children* (2006), Philip Kitcher, *The Lives to Come* (1996), Michael Sandel, *The Case Against Perfection* (2007), Allen Buchanan et al., *From Chance to Choice* (2000),

Jürgen Habermas, *The Future of Human Nature* (2003), and John Harris, *Enhancing Evolution* (2007); and Francis Fukuyama uses the word *feminism* literally twice in *Our Posthuman Future* (2002). This trend continues in essays and articles written by these same authors and other heavyweights of analytic philosophy. Unless my preliminary investigation is completely skewed, this is the norm in philosophical discussions of bioethics in genetic enhancement and selection. With a couple of important exceptions, there are few sustained interventions into this discourse by feminist philosophers. The most notable feminist contributions to the debates are perhaps those of Mary Briody Mahowald and Laura Purdy, both of whom are informed by Rawlsian liberal theory supplemented by feminist standpoint theory, and neither of whom are mentioned in the long list of texts I just cited, nor in texts that do discuss feminism in general, such as Ronald Green's *Babies by Design* (2007) and John Robertson's *Children of Choice* (1994). For an extended version of this feminist argument, see my "Whose Body, Whose Choice?" (2010).

6. For a discussion of Habermas and Derrida on cloning, see Mendieta 2003. For a discussion of Derrida and genetic engineering, see Johnson 2011.

7. Eduardo Mendieta (2003) discusses Habermas's arguments against cloning in relation to the notion of man being created in the image of God. He uses Derrida as a lens through which to read Habermas.

8. For discussions of Derrida's deconstruction of naturalism versus constructivism, see Clough 2000, Naas 2006, 2009, and 2012, Kowalksy 2012, and Zefuss 2002.

9. For discussions of Derrida's concept of *event*, see Michael Marder 2009 and 2009a. See also Shaoling 2009. For a sustained discussion of Derrida and Deleuze on the event, see Lawlor 2003.

10. Derrida says: "But whenever the one who or which remains to come does come, I am exposed, destined to be free and to decide, to the extent that I cannot foresee, predetermine, prognosticate. . . . If I know what it is necessary to decide, I do not decide. Between knowledge and decision, a leap is required, even if it is necessary to know as much and as well as possible before deciding. But if decision is not only under the authority of my knowledge but also in *my power*, if it is something 'possible' for me, if it is only the predicate of what I am and can be, I don't decide then either. That is why I often say, and try to demonstrate, how 'my' decision is and ought to be the *decision of the other* in me, a 'passive' decision, a decision of the other that does not exonerate me from any of my responsibility" (2004, 53).

11. Patrick O'Connor's analysis (2010) of Derrida's deconstruction of morality and community is interesting in this regard.

12. For discussions of Derrida's notion of interruption, see Bennington, who argues that Derrida's work interrupts the traditional domains of ethics,

politics, and literature (2000; see also Bennington 2010). See also Pirvolakis 2010, especially the section entitled "Secret Singularities," where he says: "On account of his insistence on the necessary possibilities of non-presence, secrecy, and even death, Derrida accords some primacy to discontinuity and interruption. For singular responsibility and truthful speech to be worthy of their name, and this is a demand taking place here and now, they have to presuppose a discontinuity with a preexisting order of ethical or linguistic rules. This temporal configuration interrupts the homogeneous horizon of univocity and ethical behavior opened up by the Idea. Strangely enough, precisely because this interruption disrupts horizontal continuity and progressiveness, it safeguards the status of the Idea as *infinitely* removed and unrealizable. The infinity of the Idea depends on the radical interruption of the forward movement of teleology, and the possibility of such an interruption is supplied by Derrida's thinking of the required possibility of non-presence" (137).

13. Compare the passage where Derrida says, "[I]f we examine closely the concept of cloning—the reproduction of two identical individuals, two identical structures of living beings—this has always existed; it occurs all the time in reproduction in general. Reproduction in general cannot be controlled or forbidden; we cannot deny that something identical is always returning and multiplying. The identical returns all the time. In one way or another, whether in the family, in language, in the nation, in culture and education, in tradition, one seeks to reproduce by giving oneself alibis. Without an identifying reproduction there won't be any culture either" (2004, 54). And further, when he says, "There have always been phenomena of reproduction, of the articulation between the machine and the living being" (57).

14. For discussions of Derrida's notion of *différance*, see Cheah 2009, Clough 2000, Hurst 2008, Johnson 2011, Rottenberg 2006, and Weber 2005, among many others.

2. ARTIFICIAL INSEMINATION: DECONSTRUCTING *CHOICE* VERSUS *CHANCE*

Thanks to Elissa Marder for helpful comments on an early version of this chapter. Her book *The Mother in the Age of Mechanical Reproduction* (2012) is an insightful and fascinating elaboration of the uncanniness and uncertainty inherent in the maternal function.

1. A *New York Times* columnist has written, "You can shop for gametes the way you'd go shopping for a house or a car—buying ova from an Ivy League undergraduate, or sperm from a 6-foot-8 athletic, blue-eyed Dane. The person selling you the right to bear and rear their biological offspring can do so anonymously, with no future strings attached at all. The result is a free-wheeling fertility marketplace whose impact on American life keeps increasing.

Sperm donations generate between 30,000 and 60,000 conceptions every year, and roughly 6,000 children are conceived through egg donation annually as well. About a million American adults, if not more, are the biological children of sperm donors" (Douthat 2010).

2. What the gestational carrier contributes to the developing fetus is the subject of debate amongst biologists. Certainly, the gestational carrier contributes nutrients that affect its development.

3. For an interesting discussion of what counts as motherhood and fatherhood in relation to the United Kingdom's Human Fertilization and Embryology Act, see Strathern 2011.

4. Although as always, Derrida's thinking is subtle and engages with various philosophical and literary texts, the roots of his analysis revolve around these sorts of questions: How is it possible to take the material world, the traditions, the culture, and the language into which we are born, which we are given, and make something new out of them? If we succeed, don't we also have to acknowledge a debt to those institutions out of which we come, to the past, to our parents, as it were? And if we do, if we see it coming, then in what sense is it new? This seems to be the spirit of the paradox of invention, newness, or the other that Derrida invokes.

5. For an insightful discussion of the place of the signature and proper name in Derrida's work, see Naas 2003 and 2008. In *Derrida from Now On* (2008), Naas also discusses the relationship between the father and the mother. His interpretation of why Derrida cannot name a philosophical mother in the movie *Derrida* by Amy Kofman is especially interesting (see 2008, ch. 10).

6. We might say that Derrida's *mama's boys* are those legitimate-bastard sons whose identifications with their mothers not only threaten to undermine their proper inheritance, but also put on display an ambivalence toward the mother that leads to both matricide and idealization. For example, see his discussion of Nietzsche in "Otobiographies," in *The Ear of the Other* (1985), or of Kant or Genet in *Glas* (1986). Indeed, Derrida himself imagines signing in the name of the mother as an affirmation of life, of her life, without matricide: "je veux vouloir un renoncement actif et signé à l'écriture, une vie réaffirmée. Donc sans matricide" ("La Veilleuse," 2001, 32). But this writing without matricide would also be a writing without a writing, or another sort of writing—perhaps a writing to come?

7. For fascinating discussions of the connection between the mother and death that engages Derrida, see Marder 2009 and 2010.

8. For an interesting discussion of the concept of origin in Derrida's early work, see Bennington 2010, especially "Write, He Wrote" and "Beginnings and Ends."

9. For a fascinating discussion of the "life of deconstruction," see Bennington 2010, "That's Life, Death." For a sustained analysis of Derrida on life and animals, see Lawlor 2007.

10. For discussions of Derrida's critical engagement with psychoanalysis and Freud, see Peggy Kamuf, who describes four ways in which Derrida puts pressure on psychoanalysis (2010); Elissa Marder, who uses Derrida to develop a notion of the maternal function that challenges psychoanalytic accounts of the maternal, especially in relation to mourning (2012); Michael Naas, who analyzes the relationship between photography and psychoanalysis in Derrida's writing (2011); Jeffrey Powell, who engages Freud and Derrida on the issue of justice and doing justice to Freud (2011); Elizabeth Rottenberg, who engages Derrida and Freud on dreams and mysticism (2006); Nicholas Royle, who focuses on irony in Derrida's work to show the political consequences of his engagement with psychoanalysis, among other things (2006); Andrew Ryder, who discusses Freud and Derrida in terms of the death of the father and ethics (2011); and the essays in Gabriele Schwab's edited collection *Derrida, Deleuze, Psychoanalysis* (2007).

11. This sense of invention assumes an illusory sense of our own sovereignty that falls under Derrida's deconstructive gaze most forcefully in *The Beast and the Sovereign*, to which I will return in later chapters.

3. GIRL POWERED: POETIC MAJESTY AGAINST SOVEREIGN MAJESTY

1. Bella Swan is the protagonist of Stephenie Meyer's *Twilight* books and the blockbuster movies based on them. The first film, *Twilight* (2008), stars Kristin Stewart as Bella. Bella is a high-school girl who moves to Forks, Washington to live with her father. There she meets a family of vampires and falls in love with one of them, the eternally teenaged Edward. Her best friend Jacob, who is also in love with her, is a Native American and a werewolf. Eventually Edward has to change Bella into a vampire to save her life, after which she needs to hunt wild animals for food. Suzanne Collins's *The Hunger Games* is even more popular. This book trilogy is also being made into a series of movies, the first of which, *The Hunger Games* (2012), is currently the highest-grossing film in history, with the highest-grossing opening week (eclipsing *Twilight: Eclipse*, now in second place). The protagonist is teenager Katniss Everdeen, who learned to hunt from her father before he was killed in a mining accident. Her mother and sister rely on her to provide food for the family. When her sister is chosen by lottery to participate in the fight to the death called the Hunger Games, Katniss volunteers in her stead. Her grit, determination, and level head get her through the games and lead to her victory, which culminates in her killing several mutant wolves before threatening double

suicide with her fellow District 12 contestant Peeta. Actress Jennifer Lawrence plays Katniss in the films.

2. Hanna (played by Saorise Ronan) is the sixteen-year-old protagonist of the 2011 film *Hanna*, directed by Joe Wright; screenplay by Seth Lockhead and David Farr. Hanna is raised by her father, an ex-CIA agent, in the frozen wilderness and trained as a hunter and an assassin. When she turns sixteen, he allows her to leave and sets her on a mission to kill the CIA agent responsible for the death of Hanna's mother.

3. For a fascinating discussion of the figure of the girl in Proust and Derrida, see Cixous 2007. There, Cixous suggests that while Proust pursues girls, "every passing girl," in vain, Derrida suffers from the girl.

4. For more general discussions of Derrida's theory of representation and mimesis, see Hobson 2002, Norris 1987, and Ronai 1999.

5. For a discussion of the marionette in terms of Derrida's "Faith and Knowledge," see Naas 2009 and 2012. In these studies Naas sets out Derrida's theses that science and religion have the same source and are in an autoimmune relationship.

6. For the quotation, the translator of *The Beast and the Sovereign* uses the Glenn translation of "The Meridian" that appears as an appendix to Derrida's *Sovereignties in Question: The Poetics of Paul Celan*, 3rd ed., edited by Thomas Dutoit and Outi Pasanen (New York: Fordham University Press, 2005). It is interesting that the Waldrop translation of the same passage reads: "Art, you will remember, is a puppet-like, iambic, five-footed thing without—and this last characteristic has its mythological validation in Pygmalion and his statue—without offspring" (Celan 2003, 37).

7. For discussions of the visor effect, see chapters 6 and 7.

8. For a discussion of *poesis* in Derrida's ethics, especially in relation to Heidegger, and the "mechanics of deconstruction," see Hansen 2000, especially chapter 5. For another discussion of Derrida on technology in relation to Heidegger, see Crowley 1991. Barker 1991 also talks about *poesis* and technology in Derrida, along with Benjamin and Nietzsche. Crowell 1990 offers a Heideggerian criticism of Derrida on technology.

9. The exclusion of women from fraternal politics is a central theme of Derrida's *Politics of Friendship* (1994). Many others have commented on this work in terms of its feminist implications and limitations. For example, see Deutscher 1998, Morris 2007, Perpich 2005, and Spivak 2005. Morris is especially critical of Derrida's discussion of gender: "One cannot help but observe that it is in the relative effacement of labor in the analysis of capital that Derrida's limitations as a thinker of gender become most transparent. There is a great deal in Derrida's writings about matters of sexual difference—from the erotic play of *The Post Card* (1987a), to the question of heritability

within the Abrahamic tradition in *Circumfession* (1993a), to the problematizing of the fraternal in *The Politics of Friendship* (1997), and the rethinking of the feminine 'chora' as a dimension of writing in *Khôra* (1993b). But the concern with sexual difference never generates an analysis of the labor of women, as opposed to the (conceptual or structural) labor of the feminine. A full assessment of Derrida's thought would have to account for this, just as it would have to account for the fact that, despite the enormous conceptual investment made by Derrida in the idea of auto-immunity, he almost never mentions AIDS or pharmaceutical capital (another significant factor in the realignment of state sovereignty under neoliberalism)—even as a figure of catastrophe. This spectralizing, of women and those afflicted with HIV, must necessarily haunt anthropologists who are otherwise moved by Derrida's effort to reclaim from Marx's ghost, as from religion, the aspiration to justice" (2007, 366).

10. Rottenberg tells the story of her colleagues on the translation team suggesting that there is a "grandmaw" in Little Red Riding Hood, who might say "My, what bêtises you have!" (2011, 183).

5. ELEPHANT AUTOPSY: OPTIC MACHINERY AND THE SCALE OF SOVEREIGNTY

1. For a discussion of *autopsia* in relation to Derrida's *The Animal that Therefore I Am*, see Feldman 2010. See also Marius Timmann Mjaaland's *Autopsia: Self, Death, and God after Kierkegaard and Derrida*, translated by Brian McNeil (Berlin and New York: Walter de Gruyter, 2008).

2. Marin painstakingly details and analyzes the ways in which Louis XIV's historian, Pellisson, both got his job and anticipated the necessity of painting a portrait of the king as sovereign while hiding the rhetorical flourishes necessary to do so. Marin shows how Pellisson (in a letter to the king's secretary Colbert) ingratiates himself to the king by suggesting a sort of pre-posthumous eulogy that will be read as history rather than as flattery. In other words, political rhetoric will be read or heard as historical fact. Marin argues that this operation is not unique to Pellisson or to Louis XIV, but rather is essential to the workings of sovereign power. Moreover, by analyzing the operations of power inherent in this "official aesthetic," we also learn something about the structure of representation itself, what Marin calls the "double trap" (1988, 42).

Like Derrida, throughout his work Marin is concerned with the *re* in representation and how substitution takes the place of the thing, what Derrida calls "the logic of supplementarity." Opposing the idea that the thing creates its reflection in the image or the representation, both Derrida and Marin show how the structure or logic of representation entails the inverse: the reflection or the image creates the thing as seen. In the words of Marin, "To represent, I have said, is to make the dead man come back as if he were present and living, and it is also to redouble the present and to intensify presence in the institution of a subject of representation" (1988, 7). Representation not only makes what is absent appear as present, but also authorizes the subject as the one who sees it. This is the double trap. The image appears as the thing, even more powerful than the thing insofar as it shows or tells the truth about the thing, and the subject of seeing or knowing this truth is authorized through the same operation. This is why, as Marin claims, it is in the interests of power to appropriate representation; and "representation and power share the same nature" (1988, 6). In order to secure absolute sovereignty, the sovereignty of monarchy or totalitarianism, it is necessary, then, to appropriate absolutely representations of power and monarchy.

In his analysis of the king's portrait, Marin links the dynamics of both power and representation with history as eulogy and the memorialization of the sovereign's greatness that appropriates the past and the future into an eternal monument to his sovereignty. The king needs his historian, his witness, to testify to his greatness, which is what will have made him great: "the subject of representation, to realize itself as the subject of absolute power—the absolute monarch—will be produced as the effect of narrative representation, of narrative, and of the narrative of history, where it is constructed, in the present of the prince's extraordinary act itself, the memorial of the memory of the king, a memorial that completes time in a past that is an eternalized present" (Marin 1988, 8). First, Marin states that the subject of absolute power is produced as an effect of the sovereign's representation. Second, he says that this representation is presented as a narrative history of the king's acts. Third, he suggests that this narrative operates as a memorial or monument. Finally, he argues that this memorial completes the past and turns it into an eternal present. The king's historian, then, produces the king as His Majesty the Absolute Subject through his narrative as memorial. This claim has several important ramifications for thinking about both political power or sovereignty and representation. Moreover, the lessons we learn from Marin's analysis of the king's sovereignty also apply to the sovereignty of the subject more generally, the "I" of the "I can."

What this complex analysis suggests is that we must imagine the king already dead and that his pre-posthumous eulogy produces his sovereignty as the Absolute Subject. All of the king's past actions are memorialized such that they become the eternal deeds of an eternal king. But it is not just the past that becomes part of this eternal present; rather, the future must become part of it too. For the future death of the king is already assumed, and his history is what is written for posterity. Perhaps more importantly, the king needs a witness to his greatness. The king's historian produces the king-effect through his narrative. Yet, as Marin makes plain, this narrator must efface himself from the narrative for the sake of history. In other words, this must not be the story of one man, even or especially the king's confidant, but of History itself. The narrative must be the God's-eye-view of the king. The narrative must be from the point of view of the Eternal Absolute Sovereign. This so-called history, then, is always already theological in that it assumes both an eternal, Godly point of view—that of the omniscient but absent narrator—and an Absolute Subject ordained by the history/Him.

Derrida continues to follow Marin, saying, "[H]ere it is the same thing and Marin does not fail to recall this 'asymmetry,'" and then he quotes a long passage in which Marin argues that although the king's historian adopts the absolute viewpoint in relation to the king, that does not make the historian the subject of the gaze and the king its object. Marin says, "[O]ne would be wrong to think that this position puts in return the king into the position of a seen object. In truth it is the opposite. This position is only what it is by being under the gaze of the king, in the optical cone of his eye. . . . Asymmetrical reciprocity of eyes and gaze, of eyes that see what the king does, says and thinks, and of the gaze that makes them see what he does, says, and thinks: perfect representation without excess or loss in this play of reflections or recognition, in spite of the double polarity of the historical agent and the narrator, but which operates its effects only at the price of the simulation of this spectacle" (quoted in Derrida 2009, 293). Because the narrator makes himself disappear into the omniscient voice of History itself, the eternal agency of that viewpoint is transferred onto the king as the absolute seer with the entire world falling under his gaze. The authority of God and God's view is transferred onto the king, his earthly representative, the only one authorized to see without being seen, to perform the ultimate autopsy that freezes everything under his gaze in the name of absolute knowledge.

Derrida emphasizes the collusion between sovereignty and theology throughout the history of political philosophy, wherein either explicitly or implicitly, justifications for state power and sovereignty are founded in appeals to an absolute sovereign, God. Elsewhere he insists, "It is necessary to deconstruct the concept of sovereignty, never to forget its theological filiation and to be ready to call this filiation into question wherever we discern its effects" (2004, 92). Discussing Marin's theory of the three bodies of the king, what Marin calls the "three formulas" for power or the "three entrances" of the king, Derrida parts ways slightly to suggest that the sacramental body legitimated by God is the "place of exchange, the pact or alliance" between all three (2009, 295). While this may be the case, for his part, Marin emphasizes that the sacramental power of the image as monument, whether in words or paint, "is also and indissolubly a narrative and historical representation" insofar as "the portrait as sacramental body of the king operates the historical body represented in the political symbolic body and lifts the historical body of his absence and imaginary in the symbolic fiction of the political body." Marin concludes, "The body of the king is thus visible in three senses: as sacramental body it is visibly *really present* in the visual and written currencies; as historical body it is visible as *represented*, absence become presence again and again in 'image'; as political body it is visible as *symbolic fiction signified* in its name, right, and law" (1988, 13; emphasis in original).

3. Re-presentation and re-production operate through revealing and concealing the death of the very thing they supposedly present as living. This is the paradox of representation and of testimony. As Marin's analysis makes clear, this paradox of representation is further complicated in the case of the king insofar as the king's portrait not only anticipates the king's death, such that all representations of the king are of a dead rather than living king, but also his historian and portrait painter must die too in the act of turning the first-person account into a third-person one. In other words, there can be no "I" in the king's performance of sovereignty. Or, more precisely, his "I" must be reported by a third party who hides himself; and it is this third party who is truly the bearer of the visor effect that produces the illusion of the king's sovereignty. He is the bearer of the gaze that must not be seen seeing and yet must testify to his privileged seeing as no other.

4. This position appeals to a God's-eye-view of an omniscient narrator who thereby confers omniscience on the king himself. Indeed, as Derrida argues, all testimony finds its ultimate guarantee in God, insofar as the oath or pledge to tell the truth is always sworn before God: "As God is my witness"; "So help me God."

We see this same appeal operating today not only in our courtrooms, but also in the political rhetoric of sovereign heads of state; and not only in their appeals to God or Allah, who is supposedly on their sides in holy wars on various fronts, but also in their appeals to History, from which vantage point their actions of today will be absolved or proven right in some indeterminate future, or more precisely, in the absolute future of the Last Judgment (cf. Derrida 2002a, 82). For example, in his famous prison speech of 1953, Cuba's Fidel Castro appealed to history to absolve him of the deaths resulting from his attack on the Batista regime: "La historia me absolverá." And both former British Prime Minister Tony Blair and former U.S. President George W. Bush claimed that "[h]istory will prove me right" when responding to criticisms over invading Iraq. Even President Obama continues to talk of America "winning the future" and of making the obligatory appeals to God necessary for that victory. This future with its history not only assumes an absolute judgment of God, but is also a future wherein the heads of state making such proclamations are dead. They can be absolved or proven right only after death; and their performance of the legitimation of sovereignty with appeals to God and History already assume a future without them, the future in which they will be judged right by the supreme sovereign and judge himself.

Derrida argues that all sovereign power, particularly the sort justified within the history of political philosophy, ultimately comes back to the authority or sovereignty of God. But, insofar as God is neither immediately present nor visible, nor can he be seen with one's own eyes, the foundation of sovereignty is always an absent one. And the king's or sovereign's authority is established through either an implicit or explicit appeal to this transcendent authority, ultimately based on faith and the mechanics of theology. The king or sovereign inherits the eternal "body" of God as what Marin identifies as one of the king's three bodies, a triad that produces sovereign power.

5. The three bodies and three autopsies they entail are the dynamic at the heart of the opposition between the beast and the sovereign, between animal and man and the globalization of the autopsic model of sovereignty. Derrida lists the features of this model:

> [T]he objectifying inspection of a knowledge that precisely inspects, sees, looks at the aspect of a *zōon* the life and force of which have been neutralized either by death or by captivity, or quite simply by ob-jectification that exhibits there before, to hand, before the gaze, and de-vitalizes by simple objectification, a learned objectification in the academic service of a learned society, certainly, but a society for which, between the autopsic seeing of theoretical knowledge and the autopsic seeing of the theatrical spectacle . . . the passage and transfer are more than tempting, in truth organized and institutionalized, whence the two other senses of *autopsia*: that of the necropsic relation to the cadaver and that of participation in divine power. (2009, 296)

6. In her commentary on a shorter version of the next chapter at the Spindel Conference entitled "Derrida and the Theologico-Political: From Sovereignty to the Death Penalty" (Memphis University, September 29–October 1, 2011), Elissa Marder indicated this connection between the elephant and the big man.

7. Another aspect of what Marin calls the "double trap" of sovereignty that becomes central to Derrida's analysis is the circulation of sovereign power from the king to his portrait to the viewer of the portrait. This transfer of sovereignty from the Absolute Seer, possessor of the gaze, to the one who sees (or reads, or hears) His Majesty's image (in narrative or in portraiture) follows a complex logic of making the one who sees the king seeing feel like the true seer; in other words, it makes the viewer of the image of the Royal Subject, whose gaze covers everything, a subject/object for His subject to look upon, but only indirectly, but also and thereby sharing in His power. Sovereign power circulates through the image and its illusion of immediacy from the absent king to the viewing subject, who is now both subject to and by the king's gaze. Following Marin,

Derrida recounts this paradoxical circuit of royal representation: "[T]his is a paradox, by giving the reading or watching subject of the narrative representation the illusion of himself pulling sovereignly the strings of history or of the marionette, the mystification of representation is constituted by this simulacrum of a true transfer of sovereignty. . . . He participates in sovereignty, a sovereignty he shares or borrows" (2009, 289–90).

8. For an excellent analysis of Derrida's notion of autoimmunity, see Naas 2008.

9. For a provocative discussion of mourning in Derrida in relationship to feminism, see Ziarek 2006.

10. Isabel Bradshaw claims that "a zoo called a well-known, nonhuman animal communicator to consult with their elephants because of similar [aggressive, disruptive] irregular behavior. In conversation with the elephants, the consultant learned that a resident elephant who had died was removed before the remaining elephants could mourn the body of their dead companion of many years (Varble, 2001; Khury, 2002). When the skull of the deceased was brought back to the elephant group, the elephants immediately gathered around and began a ritual of touch and caressing. . . . Thereafter the elephants resumed 'normal' behavior" (Bradshaw 2004, 149).

11. See Delight Makers Foundation, http:/delightmakers.com/news-bleat/wild-elephants-gather-inexplicably-mourn-death-of-elephant-whisperer/. Accessed May 16, 2012. See also Waterworth 2012.

12. See Bradshaw and Shore 2007; O'Connell-Rodwell 2011; McComb et al. 2001; Highfield 2006; Bradshaw 2004; Bekoff 2009; and Siebert 2011.

13. For an argument about the significance of proper names (or lack therefore) in relation to animals, see Lawlor 2007.

14. "After the death, family members show signs of grief and exhibit ritualistic behavior" (Siebert 2011, 52).

15. In parts of Asia, the Asian Elephant Specialist Group is using captive elephants to defuse tensions between humans and wild elephants (see Riddle 2007, 47–48). In China, the government is offering "dinner halls" for wild elephants in the hopes of luring them away from farms (Riddle 2007, 65).

16. Siebert reports that studies show that when young males do not have older role models, and they have been traumatized, they exhibit aggressive behavior. But if older males are reintroduced into the herd, they stop their aberrant behavior (Siebert 2011, 55).

17. "By Force of Mourning," published in *The Work of Mourning*, is one of Derrida's most powerful engagements with mourning. Following Marin's own arguments, in the eulogy Derrida locates the dynamic of the image in death and more particularly in mourning (2001c, 149). Mourning confers upon the image "its power and an increase in intensive force" (149). This power does not wait

for death; rather, as we have seen, it is conferred by the portrait of the king pre-posthumously: "the power of the image as the power of death does not wait for death, but is marked out in everything—and for everything—that awaits death: the death of the king gets its efficacity from the portrait made before the death of the king, and every image enacts its efficacity only by signifying the death from which it draws all its power" (Derrida 2001c, 151–52). The scene or spectacle of power produces power; and without it, there is no power; power does not exist in itself.

18. For an insightful analysis of this inversion of the gaze in mourning, see Saghafi 2010.

19. For an extended discussion of the figure of the ghost and phantom in Derrida, see Saghafi 2010. See also J. Hillis Miller, especially 2009, ch 4. See also Applebaum 2009, Laurence 2011, Cixous 2007, and Wood 2009.

20. For an insightful discussion of the animal's refusal in Heidegger, see Suen 2012.

21. Cf. Dennett 1991 on the mind as a Cartesian theater.

6. DEADLY DEVICES: ANIMALS, CAPITAL PUNISHMENT, AND THE SCOPE
OF SOVEREIGNTY

1. Derrida challenges this traditional belief, shared by Heidegger, that only humans die, that only *we* are capable of mourning, and only *we* perform rituals of mourning and bury our dead (cf. Derrida 2011, 41). As I mentioned in the last chapter, Derrida quotes the character Leopold Bloom from Joyce's *Ulysses* saying that only man mourns and buries his dead. Derrida clearly thinks it an error to deny death, properly speaking, mourning, or burial among animals. See also Derrida's *Of Spirit: Heidegger and the Question* (1989) and *The Animal that Therefore I Am* (2008).

2. Derrida challenges Heidegger's opposition between dying and perishing in *Of Spirit*, *The Animal that Therefore I Am*, and *The Beast and the Sovereign*, vol. 2.

3. In light of this analysis, we might wonder, however, *who* can be executed, assassinated, or murdered. Enemies of the state killed in war don't count. And neither do leaders of terrorist organizations, such as Osama Bin Laden, who was seemingly killed in cold blood; but none of the media refer to his death as murder or assassination. Who, then, can be assassinated? And what of the fact that Bin Laden's body was hidden from the media spectacle that confers sovereignty? Has President Obama's administration realized the strategy of circumventing the spectacle in order to undercut the power of the dead "king"? Derrida's analysis of the death penalty and of the machineries of death that produce different kinds of death forces us to consider what counts as a death

penalty, or murder, or assassination. It forces us to ask how various individuals and groups of people are targeted, even hunted like animals, or slaughtered like animals. And it makes us wonder what it means to be treated like an animal, to die like a dog instead of like a man.

7. DEATH PENALTIES: ETHICS, POLITICS, AND THE UNCONSCIOUS OF SOVEREIGNTY

1. Recently there has been a lot of work on Derrida and the death penalty in anticipation of the publication of his seminar on that topic. See especially Kamuf 2010 and 2010a, Naas 2011, and the Spindel Supplement: Derrida and the Theologico-Political: From Sovereignty to the Death Penalty, *Southern Journal of Philosophy* 50, issue supplement s1 (September 2012).

2. See Grimm and Grimm, 1838. These connotations continue into Modern German derivatives of *Pflicht* such as *Verpflichten*, which also means to pledge or bind in the sense of creating a social or legal bond between people.

3. Responsibility, n., in *OED*, 3rd ed., March 2010; online version September 2011,   http://www.oed.com.proxy.library.vanderbilt.edu/view/Entry/163862, accessed 19 September 2011. For etymologies of the French word *responsabilité*, see Jean-François Féraud, *Dictionnaire critique* (1787–1788), Centre National de Ressources Textuelles et Lexicales, http://dictionnaires.atilf.fr/dictionnaires/FERAUD/index.html, accessed 19 September 2011; and Walter Albardier and Philippe Genuit, *Glossaire* (Toulouse: CRIAVAS, 2010), http://www.artaas.org/documentation/oglossaire3.pdf, accessed 19 September 2011.

4. For insightful discussions of hospitality in Derrida's work, see Naas 2003, especially ch. 9, and Naas 2008, ch. 1. For a sustained analysis of the ethics of hospitality, see Still 2010. Critchley 1992 and 1999 and Duncan 2001 compare Derridean ethics with Levinasian ethics of hospitality. For a discussion of Derrida's debt to Levinas, see also Llewelyn 2002.

5. For discussions of Derrida on the issue of responsibility, see Attridge 2011, Gratton 2009, Keenan 1997, Lawlor 2002, and Llewelyn 2002.

6. For a discussion of Derrida's deconstruction of morality, especially Christian morality, see O'Connor 2010. Although O'Connor does not mention Habermas, he gives an interesting interpretation of Derrida on community that provides a nice counterpoint to Habermasian communitarianism.

7. Derrida also talks about the guillotine in *For What Tomorrow*; see especially 142–43.

8. Outside of the United States, only some Caribbean countries impose the death penalty, although for the past decade, very few, if any, prisoners have been executed.

Agamben, Giorgio. 2004. *The Open: Man and Animal*. Translated by Kevin Atell. Stanford: Stanford University Press.

Applebaum, David. 2009. *Jacques Derrida's Ghost: A Conjuration*. New York: State University of New York Press.

Aristotle. 2005. *Physics I–IV*. Translated by P. H. Wicksteed. Loeb Classical Library. Cambridge, Mass.: Harvard University Press.

Attridge, Derek. 2004. *The Singularity of Literature*. New York: Routledge.

———. 2007. "The Art of the Impossible?" In *The Politics of Deconstruction: Jacques Derrida and the Other of Philosophy*, edited by Martin McQuillan. London: Pluto Press.

———. 2011. *Reading and Responsibility: Deconstruction's Traces*. Edinburgh: Edinburgh University Press.

Balke, Friedrich. 2005. "Derrida and Foucault on Sovereignty." *German Law Journal* 6, no. 1: 71–85.

Bankovsky, Miriam. 2005. "Derrida Brings Levinas to Kant: The Welcome, Ethics, and Cosmopolitical Law." *Philosophy Today* 49, no. 2: 156–70.

Barker, Stephen. 1999. "The Problematics of Techno-Prescience." *International Studies in Philosophy* 31, no. 3: 101–10.

Bass, Alan. 2006. "Spectral, Binding Interpretation." In *Interpretation and Difference: The Strangeness of Care*, 96–186. Stanford: Standard University Press.

Baze v. Rees. 2008. 553 U.S. 35.

Beauvoir, Simone de. 1989. *The Second Sex*. Translated by H. M. Parshley. New York: Vintage.

Bekoff, Marc. 2009. "Grief in Animals: It's Arrogant to Think We're the Only Animals Who Mourn." *Psychology Today*, October 29. http://www.psychologytoday.com/blog/animal-emotions/200910/grief-in-animals-its-arrogant-think-were-the-only-animals-who-mourn.

Bellis, Mary. 2011. "Biography of Thomas Edison." About.com: Inventors. http://inventors.about.com/od/estartinventors/a/Edison_Bio.htm?r=et.

Bennington, Geoffrey. 1987. *Lyotard: Writing the Event*. New York: Columbia University Press.

———. 2000. *Interrupting Derrida*. London: Routledge.

———. 2008. "For Better and for Worse (There Again . . .)." *Diacritics* 38, nos. 1–2 (Spring): 92.

———. 2010. *Not Half No End: Militantly Melancholic Essays in Memory of Jacques Derrida*. Edinburgh: Edinburgh University Press.

Bernasconi, Robert. 1987. "Deconstruction and the Possibility of Ethics." In *Deconstruction and Philosophy*, edited by John Sallis, 122–42. Chicago: University of Chicago Press.

Biesta, Gert. 2009. "Education after Deconstruction: Between Event and Invention." In *Derrida, Deconstruction, and the Politics of Pedagogy*, edited by Michael Peters and Gert Biersta, 97–114. New York: Peter Lang.

Bonner, Sarah. 2006. "Visualizing Little Red Riding Hood." Moveable Type: Journal of the Graduate Society. Department of English, University College London. www.ucl.ac.uk/english/graduate/issue/2/sarah.htm.

Bradley, Arthur. 2011. *Originary Technicity: The Theory of Technology from Marx to Derrida*. Bloomington: Indiana University Press.

Bradshaw, Isabel G. A. 2004. "Not by Bread Alone: Symbolic Loss, Trauma, and Recovery in Elephant Communities." *Society and Animals* 12, no. 2: 143–58.

Bradshaw, Isabel G. A., and Allan Schore. 2007. "How Elephants Are Opening Doors; Developmental Neuroethology, Attachment and Social Context." *Ethology* 113:426–36.

Brenner, David A. 2005. "'Torn' Between Justice and Forgiveness: Derrida on the Death Penalty and 'Lawful Lawlessness.'" In *Crime and Punishment: Perspectives from the Humanities*, edited by Austin Sarat, 109–22. Cambridge: Emerald Group Publishing Limited.

Buchanan, Allen, Dan Brock, Norman Daniels, and Daniel Wikler. 2000. *From Chance to Choice: Genetics and Justice*. Cambridge: Cambridge University Press.

Burroughs, John. 1918. "Is Nature Cruel?" *North American Review* 208, no. 75: 588–66.

Burton, Thomas. 2009. "The Hanging of Mary, A Circus Elephant." In *A Tennessee Folklore Sampler: Selected Readings from the Tennessee Folklore Society Bulletin*, edited by Ted Olson and Anthony Cavender, 219–27. University of Tennessee Press.

Butler, Judith. 2004. "Jacques Derrida." *London Review of Books* 26, no. 4 (February 19): 32.

———. 2009. "Wise Distinctions." *London Review of Books Blog*, November 20. http://www.lrb.co.uk/blog/2009/11/20/judith-butler/wise-distinctions/.

Cain, Sarah. 2011. "Pas de Loup." Review of *The Nets of Modernism: Henry James, Virginia Woolf, James Joyce and Sigmund Freud* by Maude Ellmann, and of *The Beast and the Sovereign*, vol. 1, by Jacques Derrida. *Cambridge Quarterly* 40, no. 3 (September): 282–88.

Calcagno, Antonio. 2007. *Badiou and Derrida: Politics, Events and Their Time.* Continuum Studies in Continental Philosophy. London and New York: Continuum.

Campolo, Lisa D. 1985. "Derrida and Heidegger: The Critique of Technology and the Call to Care." *Journal of the American Academy of Religion* 53, no. 3 (September): 431–48.

Caputo, John D. 1999. "Who Is Derrida's Zarathustra? Of Fraternity, Friendship, and a Democracy to Come." *Research in Phenomenology* 29: 184–98.

Cartwright, Lisa. 1992. "'Experiments of Destruction': Cinematic Inscriptions of Physiology." Special issue, "Seeing Science." *Representations* 40 (Autumn): 129–52.

Casert, Raf, and Ryan Luca. 2009. "Bolt Sets World Record in 200 Meters; Semenya Wins 800." *Washington Post*, August 21. http://www.washingtonpost.com/wp-dyn/content/article/2009/08/20/AR2009082000362.html.

Celan, Paul. 2003. "The Meridian." In *Collected Prose of Paul Celan*, translated by Rosemarie Waldrop, 37–56. New York: Routledge Press.

Cheah, Pheng, and Suzanne Guerlac, eds. 2009. *Derrida and the Time of the Political.* Durham, N.C.: Duke University Press.

Cixous, Hélène. 2006. "The Flying Manuscript." Translated by Peggy Kamuf. *New Literary History* 37, no. 1 (Winter): 15–46.

———. 2007. "Jacques Derrida as a Proteus Unbound." *Critical Inquiry* 33, no. 2: 389–423.

———. 2007a. "The Gift of the Ghost of the Beaver and the Mole." Lecture given on September 29, Shakespeare and Derrida Conference, Cardiff University.

———. 2007b. *Insister of Jacques Derrida.* Translated by Peggy Kamuf. Edinburgh: Edinburgh University Press.

———. 2008. "The Keys To: Jacques Derrida as a Proteus Unbound." Translated by Peggy Kamuf. Special issue, "'Who?' or 'What?'—Jacques Derrida." *Discourse* 30, nos. 1–2: 71–122.

Clarey, Christopher, and Gina Kolata. 2009. "Gold Awarded amid Dispute over Runner's Sex." *New York Times*, August 21. http://www.nytimes.com/2009/08/21/sports/21runner.html?pagewanted=all.

Clough, Patricia Ticineto. 2000. "The Technical Substrates of Unconscious Memory: Rereading Derrida's Freud in the Age of Teletechnology." *Sociological Theory* 18, no. 3 (November): 383–98.

Cohen, Tom, ed. 2002. *Jacques Derrida and the Humanities: A Critical Reader.* Cambridge: Cambridge University Press.

———. 2006. "Legacies of Theory; or, Grand Central Station." *Canadian Review of Comparative Literature* 33, nos. 3–4 (September–December): 246–68.

———. 2009. "Tactless—the Severed Hand of J. D." *Derrida Today* 2 (May): 1–22.

———. 2010. "The Geomorphic Fold: Anapocalyptics, Changing Climes and 'Late' Deconstruction." *Oxford Literary Review* 32 (July): 71–89.

Colebrook, Claire. 1998. "The Future-To-Come: Derrida and the Ethics of Historicity." *Philosophy Today* 42, no. 4 (Winter): 347–60.

Combs, Scott. 2008. "Cut: Execution, Editing, and Instant Death." *Spectator* 28, no. 2 (Fall): 31–41.

Critchley, Simon. 1992. *The Ethics of Deconstruction: Derrida and Levinas*. Cambridge: Blackwell.

———. 1999. *Ethics, Politics, Subjectivity: Essays on Derrida, Levinas and Contemporary French Thought*. New York: Verso.

Crowell, Steven Galt. 1990. "Text and Technology." *Man and World* 23, no. 4 (October): 419–40.

Crowley, Paul. 1991. "Technology, Truth and Language: The Crisis of Theological Discourse." *Heythrop Journal: A Bimonthly Review of Philosophy and Theology* 32, no. 3 (July): 323–39.

De Jesus, Ronald Mendoza. 2011. "Being, Sovereignty, Unconditionality: Heidegger's *Walten* in Derrida's *La bete et le souverain II*." *Mosaic* 44, no. 3 (September): 99.

De Ville, Jacques. 2009. "Rethinking the Notion of a 'Higher Law': Heidegger and Derrida on the Anaximander Fragment." *Law and Critique* 20, no. 1: 59–78.

Debrix, François. 1999. "Specters of Postmodernism: Derrida's Marx, the New International and the Return of Situationism." *Philosophy and Social Criticism* 25, no. 1 (January): 1–21.

Deleuze, Gilles. 1968. *Différence et repetition*. Paris: Presses Universitaires de France.

Dennett, Daniel. 1991. *Consciousness Explained*. Boston: Little, Brown and Co.

Derrida, Jacques. 1976. *Of Grammatology*. Translated by Gayatri Spivak. Baltimore: Johns Hopkins University Press.

———. 1978. *Writing and Difference*. Translated by Alan Bass. Chicago: University of Chicago Press.

———. 1981. *Dissemination*. Translated by Barbara Johnson. Chicago: University of Chicago Press.

———. 1981a. *Positions*. Translated by Alan Bass. Chicago: University of Chicago Press.

———. 1982. *Margins of Philosophy*. Translated by Alan Bass. Chicago: University of Chicago Press.

———. 1985. *The Ear of the Other*. Translated by Peggy Kamuf. Omaha: University of Nebraska Press.

————. 1986. *Glas*. Translated by John Leavy and Richard Rand. Omaha: University of Nebraska Press.

————. 1989. *Of Spirit: Heidegger and the Question*. Translated by Geoffrey Bennington and Rachel Bowlby. Chicago: University of Chicago Press.

————. 1993. "Circumfessions." In *Jacques Derrida*, translated by Geoffrey Bennington, 120–132. Chicago: University of Chicago Press.

————. 1993a. *Memoirs of the Blind: The Self-Portrait and Other Ruins*. Chicago: University of Chicago Press.

————. 1993b. "Who Is the Mother? Birth, Nature, Nation." Translated from the Hungarian by Jolan Bogdan. Transcription of the Inaugural Lecture at Janus Pannonius University, Pécs, Hungary, November 12.

————. 1994. *Politics of Friendship*. Translated by George Collins. New York: Verso.

————. 1994a. *Specters of Marx: The State of the Debt, the Work of Mourning, and the New International*. Translated by Peggy Kamuf. New York: Routledge.

————. 1995. "'Eating Well,' or the Calculation of the Subject." In *Points . . . : Interviews, 1974–1994*, edited by Elisabeth Weber and translated by Peggy Kamuf et al., 255–87. Stanford: Stanford University Press.

————. 1995a. *The Gift of Death*. Translated by David Wills. Chicago: University of Chicago Press.

————. 1995b. *On the Name*. Translated by David Wood. Stanford: Stanford University Press.

————. 1998. *Monolingualism of the Other; or, The Prothesis of Origin*. Translated by Patrick Mensah. Stanford: Stanford University Press.

————. 2000. *The Instant of My Death/Demeure: Fiction and Testimony*. With Maurice Blanchot. Translated by Elizabeth Rottenberg. Stanford: Stanford University Press.

————. 2001. *On Cosmopolitanism and Forgiveness*. Translated by Mark Dooley and Michael Hughes. New York: Routledge.

————. 2001a. "On Forgiveness." In *On Cosmopolitanism and Forgiveness*, translated by M. Dooley and M. Hughes, 25–60. London: Routledge.

————. 2001b. "La Veilleuse." In *James Joyce ou L'écriture matricide* by Jacques Trilling, 7–32. Belfort: Circé.

————. 2001c. *The Work of Mourning*. Edited by Pascale-Anne Brault and Michael Naas. Chicago: University of Chicago Press.

————. 2002. *Acts of Religion*. Edited by Gil Anidjar. New York: Routledge.

————. 2002a. "Faith and Knowledge: The Two Sources of 'Religion' at the Limits of Reason Alone." Translated by Samuel Weber. In *Acts of Religion*, edited by Gil Anidjar, 40–101. New York: Routledge.

———. 2002b. "Typewriter Ribbon: Limited Ink (2)." In *Without Alibi*, edited and translated by Peggy Kamuf, 71–160. Stanford: Stanford University Press.

———. 2002c. "The University Without Condition." In *Without Alibi*, edited and translated by Peggy Kamuf, 202–37. Stanford: Stanford University Press.

———. 2003. "And Say the Animal Responded?" Translated by David Wills. In *Zoontologies: The Question of the Animal*, edited by Cary Wolfe, 121–46. Minneapolis: University of Minnesota Press.

———. 2004. *For What Tomorrow . . . : A Dialogue*. With Elisabeth Roudinesco. Translated by Jeff Fort. Stanford: Stanford University Press.

———. 2005. *Paper Machine*. Translated by Rachel Bowlby. Stanford: Stanford University Press.

———. 2005a. *Rogues*. Translated by Pascale-Anne Brault and Michael Naas. Stanford: Stanford University Press.

———. 2007. *Learning to Live Finally: An Interview with Jean Birnbaum*. Translated by Pascale-Anne Brault and Michael Naas. Hoboken, N.J.: Melville House Publishing.

———. 2007a. *Psyche: Inventions of the Other*, vol. 1. Edited and translated by Peggy Kamuf and Elizabeth Rottenberg. Stanford: Stanford University Press.

———. 2008. *The Animal that Therefore I Am*. Translated by David Wills. New York: Fordham University Press.

———. 2008a. *Psyche: Inventions of the Other*, vol. 2. Edited and translated by Peggy Kamuf and Elizabeth Rottenberg. Stanford: Stanford University Press.

———. 2009. *The Beast and the Sovereign*, vol. 1. Translated by Geoffrey Bennington. Chicago: University of Chicago Press.

———. 2010. *Séminaire La bête et le souverain*, vol. 2 (2002–2003). Paris: Galilée.

———. 2011. *The Beast and the Sovereign*, vol. 2. Translated by Geoffrey Bennington. Chicago: University of Chicago Press.

Deutscher, Penelope. 1998. "Mourning the Other, Cultural Cannibalism, and the Politics of Friendship." *Differences: A Journal of Feminist Cultural Studies* 10:159.

———. 2005. *How to Read Derrida*. London: Granta Books.

Dinzelbacher, Peter. 2002. "Animal Trials: A Multidisciplinary Approach." *Journal of Interdisciplinary History* 32, no. 3 (Winter): 405–21.

Diogenes Laërtius. 1925. *Lives of the Eminent Philosophers*. Translated by Robert Drew Hicks. Loeb Classical Library.

Dixon, Robyn. 2009. "Runner Caster Semenya Has Heard the Gender Comments All Her Life." *Los Angeles Times*, August 21. http://articles.latimes.com/2009/aug/21/world/fg-south-africa-runner21.

———. 2009a. "Caster Semenya, Runner Subjected to Gender Test, Gets Hero's Welcome in South Africa." *Los Angeles Times*, August 26. http://articles.latimes.com/2009/aug/26/world/fg-africa-runner26.

Doane, Mary Ann. 2002. *The Emergence of Cinematic Time: Modernity, Contingency, the Archive*. Cambridge, Mass.: Harvard University Press.

Dominey, Craig. 2011. "Murderous Mary." The Moonlit Road: Strange Tales of the American South. http://themoonlitroad.com/murderous-mary/.

Douthat, Ross. 2010. "The Birds and the Bees (via the Fertility Clinic)." *New York Times*, May 30. http://www.nytimes.com/2010/05/31/opinion/31douthat.html.

Duncan, Diane Moira. 2001. *The Pre-Text of Ethics: On Derrida and Levinas*. New York: P. Lang.

Dutoit, Thomas. 2012. "Jacques Derrida on Pain of Death." In *The Demands of the Dead: Executions, Storytelling, and Activism in the United States*, edited by Katy Ryan, 221–34. Iowa City: University of Iowa Press.

Dworkin, Ronald. 2000. *Sovereign Virtue: The Theory and Practice of Equality*. Cambridge, Mass.: Harvard University Press

Egorova, Y., A. Edgar, and S. Pattison. 2006. "The Meanings of Genetics: Accounts of Biotechnology in the Work of Habermas, Baudrillard and Derrida." *International Journal of the Humanities* 3, no. 2: 97–103.

Ellenberger, Henri Frédéric. 1960. "Zoological Garden and Mental Hospital." *Canadian Psychiatric Association Journal* 5 (July): 136–49.

Evans, Edward Payson. 1906. *The Criminal Prosecution and Capital Punishment of Animals*. London: W. Heinemann.

"Execution of Animals for Crimes." 1860. *Auckland Star*. PapersPast. http://paperspast.natlib.govt.nz/cgi-bin/paperspast?a=d&d=AS18760202.2.12&l=mi&e=-------10--1----obenvenue+bradley--.

Fabbri, Lorenzo. 2008. *The Domestication of Derrida: Rorty, Pragmatism and Deconstruction*. Translated by Daniele Manni. New York: Continuum.

Feldman, Allen. 2010. "Inhumanitas: Political Speciation, Animality, Natality, Defacement." In *In the Name of Humanity: The Government of Threat and Care*, edited by Ilana Feldman and Miriam Ticktin, 115–50. Durham, N.C.: Duke University Press.

Fraser, Nancy. 1997. "The Force of Law: Metaphysical or Political?" In *Feminist Interpretations of Jacques Derrida*, edited by Nancy Holland. University Park: Pennsylvania State University Press.

Freud, Sigmund. [1913] 1950. *Totem and Taboo*. Translated by James Strachey. New York: Norton.

———. [1917] 1953–74. "The Taboo of Virginity." In *The Standard Edition of the Complete Psychological Works of Sigmund Freud*, edited and translated by James Strachey, 11:191–208. London: The Hogarth Press.

———. [1922] 1953–74. "The Medusa's Head." In *The Standard Edition*, edited and translated by James Strachey, 18:273–74. London: The Hogarth Press.

Fukuyama, Francis. 2002. *Our Posthuman Future: Consequences of the Biotechnology Revolution*. New York: Picador.

Gallop, Jane. 1997. "'Women' in Spurs and Nineties Feminism." In *Derrida and Feminism: Recasting the Question of Woman*, edited by Ellen K. Feder, Mary C. Rawlinson, and Emily Zakin, 7–20. New York: Routledge.

Gaston, Sean. 2005. *Derrida and Disinterest*. New York: Continuum.

———. 2006. *The Impossible Mourning of Jacques Derrida*. New York: Continuum.

———. 2009. *Derrida, Literature and War: Absence and the Chance of Meeting*. New York: Continuum.

Gaston, Sean, and Ian Maclachlan. 2011. *Reading Derrida's "Of Grammatology."* New York: Continuum.

Girgen, Jen. 2003. "The Historical and Contemporary Prosecution and Punishment of Animals." *Animal Law* 9:97–133.

Glover, Jonathan. 2006. *Choosing Children: Genes, Disability, and Design*. Oxford: Oxford University Press.

Goodrich, Peter, Florian Hoffmann, Michel Rosenfeld, and Cornelia Vismann, eds. 2008. *Derrida and Legal Philosophy*. London: Palgrave Macmillan.

Gratton, Peter. 2006. "Questioning Freedom in the Later Work of Derrida." *Philosophy Today* 50:133–39.

———. 2009. "Derrida and the Limits of Sovereign Reason: Freedom, Equality, but not Fraternity." *Telos* 148 (Fall): 141–59.

Green, Ronald. 2007. *Babies by Design: The Ethics of Genetic Choice*. New Haven: Yale University Press.

Grimm, Jacob, and Wilhelm Grimm. 1838. *Das Deutsche Wörterbuch*. University of Trier. http://germazope.uni-trier.de:8080/Projekte/DWB.

Haas, Brian. 2011. "Death Penalty Stuck in Limbo in Tennessee." *The Tennessean*, 25 April. http://timesfreepress.com/news/2011/apr/25/death-penalty-stuck-limbo-tennessee/.

Habermas. Jürgen. 2003. *The Future of Human Nature*. Translated by Hella Beister, Willam Rehg, and Max Pensky. Cambridge: Polity Press.

Haddad, Samir. 2008. "A Genealogy of Violence, from Light to the Autoimmune." *Diacritics* 38, nos. 1–2 (Spring): 121.

Hägglund, Martin. 2008. *Radical Atheism: Derrida and the Time of Life*. Stanford: Stanford University Press.

———. 2008a. "Time, Desire, Politics: A Reply to Ernesto Laclau." *Diacritics* 38, nos. 1–2 (Spring): 180.

———. 2010. "The Non-Ethical Opening of Ethics: A Response to Derek Attridge." *Derrida Today* 3, no. 2: 295–305.

———. 2011. "Radical Atheism and 'The Arche-Materiality of Time.'" *Journal of Philosophy: A Cross-Disciplinary Inquiry* 6, no. 14: 61–65.

Hamacher, Werner. 1998. "(The End of Art with the Mask)." In *Hegel after Derrida*, edited by Stuart Barnett, 105–30. New York: Routledge.

Hansen, Mark. 2000. "The Mechanics of Deconstruction: Derrida on de Man, or Poststructuralism in an Age of Cultural Studies." *Embodying Technesis: Technology Beyond Writing*. Ann Arbor: University of Michigan Press.

Harris, John. 2004. *On Cloning*. New York: Routledge.

———. 2007. *Enhancing Evolution: The Ethical Case for Making Better People*. Princeton, N.J.: Princeton University Press.

Highfield, Roger. 2006. "Elephants Show Compassion in Face of Death." *The Telegraph*, August 14. http://www.telegraph.co.uk/news/1526287/Elephants-show-compassion-in-face-of-death.html.

Hobson, Marion. 2002. "Mimesis, Presentation and Representation." In *Jacques Derrida and the Humanities: A Critical Reader*, edited by Tom Cohen, 132–51. Cambridge: Cambridge University Press.

Howells, Christina. 1998. "The Ethics and Politics of Deconstruction and the Deconstruction of Ethics and Politics." In *Derrida: Deconstruction from Phenomenology to Ethics*. Malden, Mass.: Polity Press.

Hurst, Andrea. 2008. *Derrida vis-à-vis Lacan: Interweaving Deconstruction and Psychoanalysis*. New York: Fordham University Press.

Hyland, Drew A. 2012. "Spectres of Interpretation." *Research in Phenomenology* 42, no. 1: 3.

Johnson, Christopher. 2008. "Derrida and Technology." In *Derrida's Legacies: Literature and Philosophy*, edited by Robert Eaglestone and Simon Glendinning, 54–65. New York: Routledge.

———. 2011. "Writing in Evolution, Evolution as 'Writing.'" In *Reading Derrida's "Of Grammatology*," edited by Sean Gaston and Ian Maclachlan, 91–93. London: Continuum Press.

Kaas, Leon. 2003. "Ageless Bodies, Happy Souls: Biotechnology and the Pursuit of Perfection." *New Atlantis* 1:9–28.

Kamuf, Peggy. 1996. "Derrida on Television." In *Applying—to Derrida*, edited by John Brannigan, Ruth Robbins, and Julian Wolfreys. New York: St. Martin's Press.

———. 1997. "Deconstruction and Feminism: A Repetitition." In *Feminist Interpretations of Jacques Derrida*, edited by Nancy Holland, 103–26. University Park: Pennsylvania State University Press.

———. 2006. "From Now On." *Epoché* 10, no. 2: 203–20.

———. 2009. "The Ear Who?" *Discourse* 30, nos. 1–2: 177–90.

———. 2010. "The Dawn of the Seminar." Derrida Seminars Translation Project. http://derridaseminars.org/pdfs/2010/2010%20Presentation%20Kamuf.pdf.

———. 2010a. *To Follow: The Wake of Jacques Derrida*. Edinburgh: Edinburgh University Press.

Kant, Immanuel. 1963. "Idea for a Universal History from a Cosmopolitan Point of View." In *On History*, translated by L. W. Beck, 11–26. New York: Bobbs-Merrill.

———. 1991. *Political Writings*. Edited by H. S. Reiss. Translated by H. B. Nisbet. Cambridge: Cambridge University Press.

———. 1996. *The Metaphysics of Morals*. Translated and edited by Mary Gregor. Cambridge: Cambridge University Press.

———. 1996a. "Toward Perpetual Peace: A Philosophical Sketch." In *Practical Philosophy*, translated and edited by M. Gregor, 311–52. Cambridge: Cambridge University Press.

———. 1999. *Critique of Pure Reason*. Translated and edited by Paul Guyer and Allen Wood. Cambridge: Cambridge University Press.

Keenan, Thomas. 1989. "Deconstruction and the Impossibility of Justice." *Cardozo Law Review* 11:1675.

———. 1995. "Have You Seen Your World Today?" *Art Journal* 54, no. 4: 102.

———. 1997. *Fables of Responsibility: Aberrations and Predicaments in Ethics and Politics*. Stanford: Stanford University Press.

———. 2005. "Re JD: Remembering Jacques Derrida (part 2), Drift: Politics and the Simulation of Real Life." *Grey Room* 21 (Fall): 94–111.

Kitcher, Philip. 1996. *The Lives to Come: The Genetic Revolution and Human Possibilities*. New York: Simon and Schuster.

Kofman, Sarah. 1989. "Ca Cloche." In *Derrida and Deconstruction*, edited by Hugh J. Silverman, 114. New York: Routledge.

Koshy, Susan. 2004. *Sexual Naturalization: Asian Americans and Miscegenation*. Stanford: Stanford University Press.

Kowalsky, Nathan. 2012. "Science and Transcendence: Westphal, Derrida, and Responsibility." *Zygon* 47:118.

Krell, David Farrell. 2000. *The Purest of Bastards: Works of Mourning, Art, and Affirmation in the Thought of Jacques Derrida*. University Park: Pennsylvania State University Press.

Kristeva, Julia. 1982. *Powers of Horror*. Translated by Leon Roudiez. New York: Columbia University Press. Originally published as *Pouvoirs de l'horreur* (1980).

———. 1990. "Motherhood According to Giovanni Bellini." In *Twentieth Century Theories of Art*, edited by James M. Thompson, 441–66. Ottawa: Carlton University Press. Originally published as "Maternité selon Giovanni Bellini," in *Polylogue* (1977).

———. 1991. *Strangers to Ourselves*. Translated by L. S. Roudiez. New York: Columbia University Press. Originally published as *Étrangers à nous-mêmes* (1988).

———. 2000. *The Sense and Non-Sense of Revolt*. Translated by Jeanine Herman. New York: Columbia University Press. Originally published as *Sens et non-sens de révolte* (1996).

————. 2002. *The Portable Kristeva*. 2nd ed. Edited by Kelly Oliver. New York: Columbia University Press.

————. 2006. "A Father Is Being Beaten to Death." Presented at the Dead Father Symposium, Columbia University, April 29–30. www.kristeva.fr/father.html.

————. 2009. *This Incredible Need to Believe*. Translated by Beverley Bie Brahic. New York: Columbia University Press. Originally published as *Bisogno di credere: Un punto di vista laico* (2006).

————. 2010. *Hatred and Forgiveness*. Translated by Jeanine Herman. New York: Columbia University Press. Originally published as *Le Haine et le pardon: Pouvoir et limite de la psychanalyse III* (2005).

————. 2012. *The Severed Head: Capital Visions*. Translated by Jody Gladdings. New York: Columbia University Press. Originally published as *Visions capitales* (1998).

Laclau, Ernesto. 2008. "Is Radical Atheism a Good Name for Deconstruction?" *Diacritics* 38, nos. 1–2 (Spring): 180.

Lafontaine, Céline. 2007. "The Cybernetic Matrix of 'French Theory.'" *Theory, Culture and Society* 24 (5): 27–46.

Lawlor, Leonard. 2002. *Derrida and Husserl: The Basic Problem of Phenomenology*. Bloomington: Indiana University Press.

————. 2003. *Thinking Through French Philosophy: The Being of the Question*. Bloomington: Indiana University Press.

————. 2007. *This Is Not Sufficient: An Essay on Animality and Human Nature in Derrida*. New York: Columbia University Press.

Legrand, Pierre, ed. 2009. *Derrida and the Law*. Aldershot: Ashgate.

Leitch, Vincent B. 2007. "Late Derrida: The Politics of Sovereignty." *Critical Inquiry* 33, no. 2 (Winter): 229–47.

Levinas, Emmanuel. 1985. *Ethics and Infinity: Conversations with Phillipe Nemo*. Translated by R. Cohen. Pittsburgh: Duquesne University Press.

————. 1989. "Ethics and Politics." In *The Levinas Reader*, edited by S. Hand, 289–97. Oxford: Blackwell.

————. 1998. *Otherwise than Being, or Beyond Essence*. Translated by Alphonso Lingis. Pittsburgh: Duquesne University Press.

Levine, Michael G. 2008. "Spectral Gatherings: Derrida, Celan, and the Covenant of the Word." *Diacritics* 38, nos. 1–2 (Spring): 64.

Limbu, Bishupal. 2011. "Democracy, Perhaps: Collectivity, Kinship and the Politics of Friendship." *Comparative Literature* 63:86–110.

Lippit, Akira Mizuta. 2008. "Reflections on Spectral Life." *Discourse* 30, nos. 1–2: 242–54.

Llewelyn, John. 2002. *Appositions of Jacques Derrida and Emmauel Levinas*. Bloomington: Indiana University Press.

Loisel, Gustave. 1912. *Histoire des ménageries de l'antiquité à nos jours*, vol. 2. Paris: Octave Doin et Fils, Henri Laurens.

Long, Tony. 2008. "Aug. 6, 1890: Kemmler First to 'Ride the Lightning.'" *Wired*. http://www.wired.com/science/discoveries/news/2008/08/dayintech_0806.

Longman, Jeré. 2009. "South African Runner's Sex-Verification Result Won't Be Public." *New York Times*, November 19.

Luckhurst, Roger. 1996. "(Touching On) Tele-Technology." In *Applying: to Derrida*, edited by John Brannigan, Ruth Robbins, and Julian Wolfreys. New York: St. Martin's Press.

Lucy, Niall. 2001. "Situating Technologies: Radio Activity and the Nuclear Question." In *Beyond Semiotics: Text, Culture and Technology*, 54–71. New York: Continuum.

Luke, Robert. 2003. "Signal Event Context: Trace Technologies of the Habit@online." *Educational Philosophy and Theory* 35, no. 3 (July): 333–48.

Lundquist, Caroline. 2008. "Being Torn: Toward a Phenomenology of Unwanted Pregnancy." *Hypatia* 23, no. 3 (July–September): 136–55.

Lynch, Sandra. 2002. "Aristotle and Derrida on Friendship." *Contretemps* 3 (July): 98–108.

Mahowald, Mary. 2000. *Genes, Women, Equality*. Oxford: Oxford University Press.

———. 2006. "Between Extremes: Medical Enhancement and Eugenics." *The Pluralist* 1 (Summer): 19–34.

———. 2006a. *Bioethics and Women*. Oxford: Oxford University Press.

Marder, Elissa. 2009. "The Sex of Death and the Maternal Crypt." *Parallax* 15, no. 1: 5–20.

———. 2010. "Dark Room Readings: Scenes of Maternal Photography." *Oxford Literary Review* 32 (December): 231–70.

———. 2010a. "Ewa Ziarek's Virtually Impossible Ethics." In *Recenterings of Continental Philosophy*, edited by Cynthia Willett and Len Lawlor. Selected Studies in Phenomenology and Existential Philosophy, vol. 35. Chicago: DePaul University. *Philosophy Today* 54, Supplement 2010: 51–58.

———. 2011. *The Mother in the Mechanical Age of Reproduction*. New York: Fordham University Press.

Marder, Michael. 2009. *The Event of the Thing: Derrida's Post-Deconstructive Realism*. Toronto: University of Toronto Press.

———. 2009a. "From the Concept of the Political to the Event of Politics." *Telos* 147:55–76.

Marquardt, Elizabeth. 2010. With Norval D. Glenn and Karen Clark. "My Daddy's Name is Donor: A New Representative Study of Adults Conceived Through Sperm Donation." New York: Institute for American Values.

———. 2011. "One Parent or Five? A Global Look at Today's New Intentional Families." New York: Institute for American Values.

Marin, Louis. 1988. *Portrait of the King*. Translated by Martha M. House. Minneapolis: University of Minnesota Press. Originally published as *Le portrait du roi* (1981).

———. 1990. *To Destroy Painting*. Translated by Mette Hjort. Chicago: University of Chicago Press. Originally published as *Détruire la peinture* (1977).

———. 2000. "Caravaggio's 'Head of the Medusa': A Theoretical Perspective" (from *To Destroy Painting*). In *The Medusa Reader*, edited by Marjorie Garber and Nancy J. Vickers. New York: Taylor and Francis.

Matuštík, Martin Beck. 2004. "Between Hope and Terror: Habermas and Derrida Plead for the Im/Possible." *Epoché* 9, no. 1 (Fall): 1–18.

McComb, Karen, et al. 2001. "Matriarchs as Repositories of Social Knowledge in African Elephants." *Science* 292 (April 20): 491–94.

McKeon, Richard. 1957. "The Development and the Significance of the Concept of Responsibility." *Revue Internationale de Philosophie* 11, no. 39: 3–32.

McQuillan, Martin. 2009. *Deconstruction after 9/11*. London: Routledge.

Mendieta, Eduardo. 2003. "We Have Never Been Human, or, How We Lost Our Humanity: Derrida and Habermas on Cloning." *Philosophy Today* 47, no. 5 (December 31): 168–74.

Miller, J. H. 2006. "Derrida's Remains." Special issue, "After Derrida." *Mosaic* 39, no. 3 (September): 97–211

———. 2006a. "Sovereignty Death Literature Unconditionality Democracy University." *Canadian Review of Comparative Literature* (September–December): 233–45.

———. 2008. "Derrida's Politics of Autoimmunity." *Discourse* 30, nos. 1–2: 208–25.

———. 2009. *For Derrida*. New York: Fordham University Press.

Mitchell, W. J. T., and Arnold I. Davidson, eds. 2007. *The Late Derrida*. Chicago: University of Chicago Press.

Morris, Rosalind C. 2007. "Legacies of Derrida." *Annual Review of Anthropology* 36:355–89.

Motluk, Alison. 2005. "Execution by Injection Far from Painless." *New Scientist*, 14 April. http://www.newscientist.com/article/dn7269-execution-by-injection-far-from-painless.html.

Mundy, Liza. 2007. *Everything Conceivable: How Assisted Reproduction Is Changing Our World*. New York: Random House.

Murphy, Ann V. 2010. "All Things Considered: Sensibility and Ethics in the Later Merleau-Ponty and Derrida." *Continental Philosophy Review* 42, no. 4: 435–47.

Naas, Michael. 1995. "Have You Seen Your World Today?" *Art Journal* 54, no. 4: 102.

———. 2003. "History's Remains: Of Memory, Mourning, and the Event." *Research in Phenomenology* 33:75.

———. 2003a. "Just a Turn Away: Apostrophe and the *Politics of Friendship.*" In *Taking on the Tradition: Jacques Derrida and the Legacies of Deconstruction*, 136–53. Stanford: Stanford University Press.

———. 2005. "Kurios George and the Sovereign State." *Radical Philosophy Review* 7, no. 2: 1–20.

———. 2005a. "Re JD: Remembering Jacques Derrida (part 2), Drift: Politics and the Simulation of Real Life." *Grey Room* 21 (Fall): 94–111.

———. 2006. "'One Nation . . . Indivisible': Jacques Derrida on the Autoimmunity of Democracy and the Sovereignty of God." *Research in Phenomenology* 36:15–44.

———. 2007. "Comme si, comme ça: Phantasms of Self, State, and a Sovereign God." *Mosaic* 40, no. 2 (June): 1.

———. 2007a. "Derrida's Laïcité." *New Centennial Review* 7, no. 2 (Fall): 21–42.

———. 2008. *Derrida from Now On*. New York: Fordham University Press.

———. 2009. "Miracle and Machine: Derrida's Faith." *Research in Phenomenology* 39, no. 2: 184–203.

———. 2010. "Now Smile! Recent Developments in Jacques Derrida's Work on Photography." *South Atlantic Quarterly* 110, no. 1 (Fall): 205–22.

———. 2011. "When It All Suddenly Clicked: Deconstruction after Psychoanalysis after Photography." *Mosaic* 44, no. 3 (September): 81–98.

———. 2012. *Miracle and Machine: Jacques Derrida and the Two Sources of Religion, Science, and the Media*. New York: Fordham University Press.

Nietzsche, Friedrich. [1882] 1974. *The Gay Science*. Translated by Walter Kaufmann. New York: Vintage Books.

———. 2003. *Writing from the Late Notebooks*. Translated by R. Bittner. Cambridge: Cambridge University Press.

Norris, Christopher. 1987. *Derrida*. London: Fontana.

O'Byrne. Anne. 2010. *Natality and Finitude*. Bloomington: Indiana University Press.

O'Connell-Rodwell, Caitlin. 2011. "Ritualized Bonding in Male Elephants." *New York Times*, Scientist at Work Blog, July 20. http://scientistatwork.blogs.nytimes.com/2011/07/21/ritualized-bonding-in-male-elephants/.

O'Connor, Patrick. 2010. *Derrida: Profanations*. New York: Continuum.

Ofrat, Gideon. 2001. *The Jewish Derrida*. Translated by Peretz Kidron. Syracuse: Syracuse University Press.

Oliver, Kelly. 1995. *Womanizing Nietzsche: Philosophy's Relation to "the Feminine."* New York: Routledge Press.

———. 1997. *Family Values: Subjects between Nature and Culture*. New York: Routledge Press.

———. 1998. *Subjectivity without Subjects: From Desiring Mothers to Abject Fathers*. New York: Rowman and Littlefield.

———. 2001. *Witnessing: Beyond Recognition*. Minneapolis: University of Minnesota Press.

———. 2004. *The Colonization of Psychic Space: A Psychoanalytic Social Theory of Oppression*. Minneapolis: University of Minnesota Press.

———. 2007. "Tropho-Ethics: Derrida's Homeopathic Purity." *Harvard Review of Philosophy* 15 (Fall): 37–57.

———. 2007a. *Women as Weapons of War: Iraq, Sex, and the Media*. New York: Columbia University Press.

———. 2009. *Animal Lessons: How They Teach Us to Be Human*. New York: Columbia University Press.

———. 2010. "Enhancing Evolution: Whose Body? Whose Choice?" *Southern Journal of Philosophy* 48:74–96.

———. 2012. *Knock Me Up, Knock Me Down: Images of Pregnancy in Hollywood Film*. New York: Columbia University Press.

———. 2013. "The *Slow and Differentiated* Machinations of Deconstructive Ethics." In *Blackwell Companion to Derrida*, edited by Len Lawlor. Oxford: Blackwell.

Orenstein, Catherine. 2003. *Little Red Riding Hood Uncloaked: Sex, Morality, and the Evolution of a Fairy Tale*. New York: Basic Books.

Pear, Robert. 2011. "Recession Officially Over, U.S. Incomes Kept Falling." *New York Times*, October 9. http://www.nytimes.com/2011/10/10/us/recession-officially-over-us-incomes-kept-falling.html.

Perpich, Diane. 2005. "Universality, Singularity, and Sexual Difference: Reflections on Political Community." *Philosophy and Social Criticism* 31 (June): 445–60.

Pettman, Dominic. 2010. "After the Beep: Answering Machines and Creaturely Life." *boundary 2* 37, no. 2: 133–53.

Pirovolakis, Eftichis. 2010. *Reading Derrida and Ricoeur: Improbable Encounters between Deconstruction and Hermeneutics*. New York: State University of New York Press.

Plato. 1993. *Sophist*. Translated by Nicholas P. White. New York: Hackett.

Porter, Mark. 2009. "Male or Female? It's Not So Simple." *Times* (London), August 24: A35.

Powell, Jeffrey. 2011. "Being Just with Freud . . . after Derrida." *Mosaic* 44, no. 3 (September): 133.

Prenowitz, Eric. 2008. "Crossing Lines: Jacques Derrida and Hélène Cixous on the Phone." *Discourse* 30, nos. 1–2: 123–56.

Purdy, Laura. 1996. *Reproducing Persons: Issues in Feminist Bioethics*. Ithaca: Cornell University Press.

Quiroga, Seline Szkupinski. 2007. "Blood Is Thicker than Water: Policing Donor Insemination and the Reproduction of Whiteness." *Hypatia* 22, no. 2 (Spring): 143–61.

Raffoul, François. 2008. "Derrida and the Ethics of the Im-Possible." *Research in Phenomenology* 38, no. 2: 270–90.

Renoir, Jean, director. 1939. *The Rules of the Game* (*La Règle de jeu*). Nouvelles Éditions de Films (NEF).

Ricoeur, Paul. 2000. *The Just.* Translated by D. Pellauer. Chicago: University of Chicago Press.

Riddle, Heidi. 2007. "Elephant Response Units (ERU)." *Gajah* 26:47–53.

Robertson, John. 1994. *Children of Choice: Freedom and the New Reproductive Technologies.* Princeton, N.J.: Princeton University Press.

Roffe, Jonathan. 2004. "Ethics." In *Understanding Derrida*, edited by Jack Reynolds, 37–45. New York: Continuum.

Rogers, Nicole. 2007. "Violence and Play in Saddam's Trial." *Melbourne Journal of International Law* 8:428.

Ronai, Carol Rambo.1999. "The Next Night *Sous Rature*: Wrestling with Derrida's Mimesis." *Qualitative Inquiry* 5, no. 1 (March): 114–29.

Rottenberg, Elizabeth, ed.. 2000. *Deconstructions: A User's Guide.* London: Palgrave.

———. 2006. "Jacques Derrida's Language (Bin Laden on the Telephone)." *Mosaic* 39, no. 3 (September): 173.

———. 2006a. "The Legacy of Autoimmunity." *Mosaic* 39, no. 3 (September): 1–14.

———. 2006b. "The Resistance to Interpretation." *Philosophy Today* 50: 83–90.

———. 2009. *In Memory of Jacques Derrida.* Edinburgh: Edinburgh University Press.

———. 2011. "Devouring Figures: The Last Seminars of Jacques Derrida." *Philosophy Today* 55: 177

Royle, Nicholas. 2005. "Blind Cinema." Introduction to *Derrida: Screenplay and Essays on the Film*, edited by Kirby Dick and Amy Ziering Kofman, 10–21. Manchester: Manchester University Press.

Russell, Camisha. 2010. "The Limits of Liberal Choice: Racial Selection and Reprogenetics." Special issue, "Spindel Supplement: The Sexes of Evolution." *Southern Journal of Philosophy* 48, issue supplement s1 (September): 97–108.

Ryder, Andrew. 2011. "Politics after the Death of the Father: Democracy in Freud and Derrida." *Mosaic* 44, no. 3 (September): 115.

Saghafi, Kas. 2006. "The Ghost of Jacques Derrida." *Epoché* 10 (2): 263–86.

———. 2006a. "Salut-ations." Special issue, "After Derrida." *Mosaic* 39, no. 3 (September): 151.

———. 2010. *Apparitions—Of Derrida's Other.* New York: Fordham University Press.

Sandel, Michael. 2007. *The Case against Perfection: Ethics in the Age of Genetic Engineering*. Cambridge, Mass.: Harvard University Press.

———. 2004. "The Case against Perfection: What's Wrong with Designer Children, Bionic Athletes, and Genetic Engineering." *Atlanta Monthly* 292, no. 3 (October): 50–54, 56–60, 62.

Savulescu, Julian, and Nick Bostrom, eds. 2009. *Human Enhancement*. Oxford: Oxford University Press.

Schroeder, Joan Vannorsdall. 1997. "The Day They Hanged an Elephant in East Tennessee." *Blue Ridge Country Magazine*. http://blueridgecountry.com/articles/mary-the-elephant/page-5.html.

Schwab, Gabriele, ed. 2007. *Derrida, Deleuze, Psychoanalysis*. New York: Columbia University Press.

———. 2008. "Derrida, the Parched Woman, and the Son of Man." *Discourse* 30, nos. 1–2: 226–41.

Scribner, F. Scott. 2001. "Technologies of Spirit in Plato, Derrida, and Deleuze." *Philosophical Writings* 17 (Summer): 29–41.

Segarra, Marta. 2007. "Friendship, Betrayal, and Translation: Cixous and Derrida." Special issue, "Following Derrida: Legacies." *Mosaic* 40, no. 2 (June): 91.

Seneca, Lucius Annaeus. 2011. *On Benefits* [*De Beneficiis*]. Translated by Aubrey Stewart. N.p.: Aeterna.

Seshadri-Crooks, Kalpana. 2003. "Being Human: Bestiality, Anthropophagy, and Law." *Umbr(a): Ignorance of the Law* (2003): 97–116.

Sheldrick, Daphne. 1992. "Elepant Emotion." Elephant Information Repository. http://elephant.elehost.com/About_Elephants/Stories/Real_Life_Stories/Elephant_Emotion/elephant_emotion.html.

Siebert, Charles. 2006. "An Elephant Crackup?" *New York Times Magazine*, October 8, 42–72.

———. 2011. "Orphans No More." *National Geographic*, September, 40–65.

Simmons, Laurence. 2011. "Jacques Derrida's Ghostface." *Angelaki: Journal of the Theoretical Humanities* 16, no. 1: 129–41.

Slot, Owen. 2009. "Caster Semenya Faces Sex Test before She Can Claim Victory." *Times* (London), August 20, Sport, 58.

———. 2009a. "Caster Semenya Almost Boycotted Medal Ceremony." *Times* (London), August 22, Sport, 19.

Smith, Alex Duval, and Stewart Maclean. 2009. "Fears for Caster Semenya over Trauma of Test Results." *The Observer*, September 13, Sports, 1.

Smith, Kiki. 2003. "Kiki Smith: Prints, Books and Things." Multimedia, Museum of Modern Art. www.moma.org/interactives/exhibitions/2003/kikismith/.

Sobchak, Vivian. 1984. "Inscribing Ethical Space." *Quarterly Review of Film Studies* 9, no. 4: 283–300.

Sorel, Alexandre. 1876. "Procès contre des animaux et insectes suivis au Moyen-âge dans la Picardie et le Valois." *Bulletin de la Société Historique de Compiègne* 3 (1876–1877), 269–314.

Spitzer, Anais. 2011. *Derrida, Myth and the Impossibility of Philosophy*. New York: Continuum.

Spivak, Gayatri C. 2005. *Death of a Discipline*. New York: Columbia University Press.

Srajek, Mark C. 2000. *In the Margins of Deconstruction: Jewish Conceptions of Ethics in Emmanuel Levinas and Jacques Derrida*. Pittsburgh: Duquesne University Press.

Standish, Paul. 2000. "Fetish for Effect." *Journal of Philosophy of Education* 34, no. 1 (February): 151–68.

Stiegler, Bernard. 2001. "Derrida and Technology: Fidelity at the Limits of Deconstruction and the Prosthesis of Faith." In *Jacques Derrida and the Humanities: A Critical Reader*, ed. Tom Cohen. Cambridge: Cambridge University Press.

Still, Judith. 2010. *Derrida and Hospitality: Theory and Practice*. Edinburgh: Edinburgh University Press.

Strathern, Marilyn. 2011. "What Is a Parent?" *HAU: Journal of Ethnographic Theory* 1 (1): 245–278.

Suen, Alison. 2012. "The Poverty of Kinship: Heidegger on the Human-Animal Linguistic Divide." Ph.D. dissertation, Vanderbilt University.

Thomson, A. J. P. 2005. *Deconstruction and Democracy: Derrida's Politics of Friendship*. New York: Continuum.

Trifonas, Peter Pericles, and Michael A. Peters, eds. 2005. *Deconstructing Derrida: Tasks for the New Humanities*. London: Palgrave Macmillan.

Vattimo, Gianni, and Sebastian Gurcillo. 2001. "Interpretation and Nihilism as the Depletion of Being: A Discussion with Gianni Vattimo about the Consequences of Hermeneutics." *Theory and Event* 5, no. 2.

Von Arnim, Hans, ed. 2004. *Stoicorum Veterum Fragmenta*, vols. 1 and 2. Munich: J. G. Saur Verlag. http://www.archive.org/details/stoicorumveterumo1arniuoft.

Wadiwel, Dinesh Joseph. 2010. "A Human Right to Stupidity." *Borderlands* 9, no. 3 (December). http://www.borderlands.net.au/vol9no3_2010/wadiwel_derrida .htm.

Walt, Johan. 2005. "Interrupting the Myth of the Partage: Reflections on Sovereignty and Sacrifice in the Work of Nancy, Agamben and Derrida." *Law and Critique* 16, no. 1: 277–99.

Waterworth, Tanya. 2012. "Jungle Giants Come to Bid Farewell to 'Elephant Whisperer.'" *The Star* (Johannesburg), May 10, 3.

Weber, Elisabeth. 2005. "Deconstruction Is Justice." *SubStance* 34, no. 1, issue 106: 38–43.

Weber, Samuel. 2008. "Rogue Democracy." *Diacritics* 38, nos. 1–2 (Spring): 104.

Williams, R. John. 2005. "Naked Creatures: Robinson Crusoe, the Beast, and the Sovereign." *Comparative Critical Studies* 2, no. 3 (October): 337–48.

Wood, Sarah. 2008. "Dream-hole." *Journal of European Studies* 38, no. 4: 373–82.

———. 2009. "Centre-piece." *Theory and Event* 12, no. 1.

———. 2009a. "Some Scraps on Beauty-in-the-Ghost." *Parallax* 15, no. 1: 80–89.

Young, Iris Marion. 2005. "Pregnant Embodiment." In *On Female Body Experience: "Throwing Like a Girl" and Other Essays*. New York: Oxford University Press.

Zehfuss, Maja. 2002. "The Politics of 'Reality': Derrida's Subversions, Constructivism and German Military Involvement Abroad." In *Constructivism in International Relations: The Politics of Reality*, 196–249. Cambridge: Cambridge University Press.

Ziarek, Ewa. 2001. *An Ethics of Dissensus: Postmodernity, Feminism, and the Politics of Radical Democracy*. Stanford: Stanford University Press.

———. 2006. "Encounters Possible and Impossible: Derrida and Butler on Mourning." *Philosophy Today* 50:144–55.

Zlomislic, Marko. 2007. *Jacques Derrida's Aporetic Ethics*. Lanham, Md.: Lexington Books.